How to Get Pregnant with IVF

Celebrating
30 Years of Publishing
in India

How to Get Pregnant with IVF

A Practical Guide to Fertility Treatments

GITANJALI BANERJEE

HarperCollins *Publishers* India

First published in India by HarperCollins *Publishers* 2022
4th Floor, Tower A, Building No 10, DLF Cyber City,
DLF Phase II, Gurugram, Haryana – 122002
www.harpercollins.co.in

2 4 6 8 10 9 7 5 3 1

Copyright © Gitanjali Banerjee 2022

P-ISBN: 978-93-5629-532-2
E-ISBN: 978-93-5629-533-9

The views and opinions expressed in this book are the author's own and
the facts are as reported by her, and the publishers are not in any
way liable for the same.

Gitanjali Banerjee asserts the moral right
to be identified as the author of this work.

All rights reserved. No part of this publication may be reproduced,
stored in a retrieval system, or transmitted, in any form or by any
means, electronic, mechanical, photocopying, recording or otherwise,
without the prior permission of the publishers.

Typeset in 11.5/15.2 Garamond at
Manipal Technologies Limited, Manipal

Printed and bound at
Thomson Press (India) Ltd

To the love of my life, my son, Athindra ♥
IVF-born baby

Medical Disclaimer

The information presented is the author's opinion and does not constitute any health or medical advice. The content of this book is for informational purposes only and is not intended to diagnose, treat, cure, or prevent any condition or disease. Please seek advice from your healthcare provider for your personal health concerns prior to taking healthcare advice from this book

Contents

1. Leap of Faith — 1
2. Tests, Tests and More Tests — 19
3. The Difficult Acceptance — 55
4. The Different Types of Infertility: Understand Your Type — 70
5. IUI: The First Step — 88
6. IVF: The Basics — 98
7. The Different Types of IVF and their Step-by-Step Process — 150
8. How to Prepare for IVF — 183
9. Result Day — 225
10. Male Infertility: The Elephant in the Room — 250
11. Managing Social Pressure — 277
12. When to Stop: The Road Ahead — 307

Acknowledgements — 329

A Note to the Reader

'Owning our story and loving ourselves through that process is the bravest thing that we will ever do.'

– Brene Brown

I WAS TWENTY-THREE AND FRESH OUT OF JAWAHARLAL NEHRU University, brimming with the knowledge of world politics but totally unaware of the real world when my father dropped the bombshell of an arranged marriage. With assurances of being able to pursue my PhD and career post marriage, I agreed to marry. Little did I knew life had a rollercoaster ride waiting for me.

After a customary one year of honeymoon period, the ever-pervasive question, 'So, when is the good news?' started to haunt us. Well, I naively thought, 'Let's tick this milestone out quickly and then I will be free of all societal pressures, free to pursue my dreams.'

And with this began the ten long and gruelling years of fighting infertility. Post five miscarriages, three molar pregnancies, one failed IUI, one failed IVF, and a brush with ovarian cancer, I finally found light at the end of tunnel and was successfully pregnant on second IVF attempt. I stand here in front of you to openly talk about my infertility journey.

I can never forget the pain and suffering, the loneliness, the depression and desperation, the feeling of being cut off from society, and the turmoil within during this journey. It has made me who I am today. It is a very important part of my life and my personality. There are many layers of suffering through the process of IVF—medical, physical, mental, psychological, financial, and social, all of which lead to marital discord, falling into depression, even to the extent of getting suicidal, cutting oneself off socially, and a lot of traumas. There are cycles of hope and frustration. There are choices to make. There are tough decisions to take. I have been through all that. The path to IVF is no easy task. Only the brave can tread through. And through this book, I want to salute each and every couple who is going through or has been through IVF.

Once I had my son, I started to think: 'Why was the journey so overwhelming and unmanageable? If I, an educated woman from a decent financial background, married into the Armed Forces, felt so lonely and confused, then what about those women who aren't so privileged or empowered, and how are they managing this infertility struggle? Could I have managed the treatment better? Where did I go wrong?' All these questions and more kept me awake at nights. I was constantly thinking why God had

A Note to the Reader

given me this complex journey of infertility. The seeds of Fertility Dost were sown. I had found my life's purpose.

I left my cushy corporate job as content marketer and started building India's first community and platform for couples struggling with infertility, Fertility Dost. It is here that I met so many couples, listened to so many stories, answered so many questions, calmed many nerves and handheld them towards their fertility goals. Slowly news of miraculous conception and good news from Fertility Dost community members started to pour in.

The truth behind these miracles was nothing miraculous! It is simple science, conscious lifestyle and clear mind that helps your steer past the messy situation towards love and light.

This book is a compilation of my personal journey, the fertility journeys of many couples at various stages of fertility treatments, and inputs from the IVF doctors. The unique feature of the book is that it breaks down the complete process of IVF and other fertility treatments, keeping you at the centre of it, making it easy for you to take tips, understand holistically and take well-informed decisions. It has usable, practical and simple techniques to ensure that you reach your parenthood goal hassle-free.

All the best!

1
Leap of Faith

When I was going through my fertility journey, the God I turned to most was Gopal, my baby Krishna. His wide eyes, round cheeks, his crawling stance was, to me, the purest form of innocence. He was the baby I wanted. I would sit for hours in front of him—crying, begging, even picking him up at times and getting angry with him.

Figure 1.1: My Ladoo Gopal

Source: www.shutterstock.com.

'Why won't you bless me? Why won't you come to my house? Do whatever you want but give me enough strength and dignity to deal with infertility', I'd say to him.

I couldn't let my dignity strip away gradually. I prayed all the time. But the truth was that I wasn't praying, I was begging. The funny thing is that Gopal listened to me when I stopped begging.

I didn't know it then, but the fact is that I was not alone in this abyss.

In India, nearly 27.5 million couples who are actively trying to conceive suffer from infertility.[1] Over the last few decades, a decline in fertility rates has been observed due to a higher prevalence of contraceptive use, late marriage or having kids late.[2] According to the Indian Society for Assisted Reproduction (ISAR), infertility currently affects about 10–14 per cent of the Indian population, with higher rates in urban areas where one out of six couples are impacted.[3] Globally, the World Health Organization (WHO) estimates that 60–80 million couples worldwide currently suffer from

---

1 'Call for Action: Expanding IVF Treatment in India', PDFCoffee, July 2015, available at https://pdfcoffee.com/ey-call-for-action-expanding-ivf-treatment-in-indiapdf-pdf-free.html.

2 Ibid.

3 N. Lal, 'India's Hidden Infertility Struggles: Behind India's Booming Population is Another Story: Declining Fertility Rates and Desperate Couples', The Diplomat, 30 May 2018, available at https://thediplomat.com/2018/05/indias-hidden-infertility-struggles/#:~:text=According%20to%20the%20Indian%20Society,suffer%20from%20infertility%20in%20India.

infertility.[4] Infertility varies across regions of the world and is estimated to affect 8–12 per cent of couples worldwide.[5]

It's time that we stop talking about infertility in 'hush-hush' tones. Life is not always fair, and when it is not, it is one hell of a life!

Breaking the Cycle

Anyone who is trying to have a baby will be familiar with this routine.

It starts with a trip to the gynaecologist, to whom we proudly announce that we are planning a family. The doctor will tell us the basic stuff—ovulation chart, happy hormones, and prescribe us preliminary tests, folic acid tablets, and some supplements.

Then, we have sex, diligently, as if it were homework, in that sacred time period of ten days, often to the irritation and angst of the husband because when you are told to have sex it ceases to be fun. In the movie *Good Newwz* (2020), Kareena Kapoor (who plays Akshay Kumar's wife) is trying to have a baby, so she follows the ovulation clock to a tee.

---

4 'Infecundity, Infertility, and Childlessness in Developing Countries', Comparative Reports, The Demographic and Health Surveys (DHS) Program, No. 9. Calverton, Maryland, USA: ORC Macro and the World Health Organization; 2004. World Health Organization.

5 Shireen J. Jejeebhoy, 'Looking Back, Looking Forward: A Profile of Sexual and Reproductive Health in India', Sociological Bulletin 55, no. 2 (2006) (New Delhi: Population Council; 2004), pp. 67–72, available at https://www.jstor.org/stable/23620577.

In one scene, she says, 'Do you want a baby or not?', to which Akshay Kumar replies, 'Yes, I want to have a baby but going to the bedroom shouldn't feel like we are heading for a surgical strike.' This aptly brings out the desperation and frustration of a couple trying to get pregnant.

Our hectic and stressful cosmopolitan lives don't help either. Your husband has an important meeting at work, and you keep messaging him to return home. Your romantic wait transforms into frustration and you end up having a fight with him, pushing up stress levels. Yet, you try every arrow in your quiver to coax, cajole and seduce him. You plan your life around ovulation. You follow every myth and trick in the book. You know that you should lie on your left side after sex, place a pillow underneath your hips when having sex, not wash yourself post-sex, hold your legs upright after sex, and even avoid certain foods.

Then, you wait desperately, ticking off each day on the calendar, praying that you miss your period. You keep the self-help pregnancy test kit ready but hidden somewhere beneath your clothes in the closet because you don't want to jinx it. Every month, you pray for the period to *not come*. Missing period is the most joyful event for a woman who is trying to conceive. However, the more you wish to miss your period, the more stubbornly it keeps coming back every month.

When you get your period, you cannot help but feel depressed and lost because you've lost another month of your precious biological timeline. You don't have the strength to do it all over again next month. You only have that much energy! Your husband thinks that your depression is regular pre-menstrual syndrome (PMS). And even if you muster all your strength to try and explain to him, looking for some compassion, pat comes the reply, 'Don't worry, we'll try again next month.'

But how long can you run away from the truth?

When to See a Fertility Expert?

According to the WHO, 'Infertility is "a disease of the reproductive system defined by the failure to achieve a clinical pregnancy after 12 months or more of regular unprotected sexual intercourse".'[6]

However, I do believe that there is no harm in seeing a fertility expert if you have been actively trying to get pregnant for six months or more with no luck. Especially if you live in an urban city, have a high-stress job and a not-so-yogic lifestyle, it is better to start early.

Meeting a fertility doctor at this stage does not mean that you will be pushed for in vitro fertilization (IVF) the very next month. The roadmap should look something like this:

1. Go for a fertility consultation.
2. Understand the premise of fertility treatments.
3. Get basic fertility tests done.
4. And more importantly, take this time to prepare yourself emotionally for the treatments (if required).

---

6   'Infertility', World Health Organization, 14 September 2020, available at https://www.who.int/news-room/fact-sheets/detail/infertility.

This exercise can help you prepare mentally and get a sense of the road ahead. You also save on time which is often wasted by couples simply because they wait for a year or more with a gynae.

Think about the following two roadmaps and how they impact a couple's decision to get pregnant.

Couple A

1. Consults a gynae.
2. Tries to conceive naturally for a year.
3. Waits and waits.
4. Towards the end of the year, they begin to panic.
5. In this situation of panic, anxiety and desperation with their existing gynae, they make decisions in a frenzy.
6. Now they begin to look for a fertility speciality, which will take some time. They also end up wasting more time preparing themselves mentally for this visit.
7. When they finally meet the fertility doctor, all they want are *quick results*.

Couple A is now gripped by anxiety. Wrong expectations are set due to this anxiety. And we all know that anxiety is a big roadblock to conception.

Couple B

1. Consults a gynae.
2. Tries to conceive naturally.

3. Waits for six months and then sees a fertility expert.
4. Gets basic tests done and is put on some fertility enhancement medicines.
5. Follows the treatment line.

Couple B saves time in starting the treatment line and is also less anxious because they know that they are moving in the right direction.

It is important to remember that at this stage you can go to any reputed, credited fertility specialist to get an initial opinion. I will talk in depth about how to find the right IVF doctor in Chapter 6.

Age

Age is an extremely crucial factor in pregnancy and the success of fertility treatments. Fertility in women in the age group of twenty-five to twenty-nine years is reduced on an average by 6 per cent, compared to that of women in the age group of twenty to twenty-four years, 14 per cent for women in the age group of thirty to thirty-four years, and 31 per cent for women in the age group of thirty-five to thirty-nine years, with much greater decline thereafter.[7] Basically, fertility declines with increasing age in women.

---

7 J. Menken, J. Trussell and U. Larsen, 'Age and infertility' Science 233, no. 4771(1986), pp. 1389–94, available at https://www.science.org/doi/10.1126/science.3755843.

Often, we ignore this factor because people around us misleadingly tell us, 'Oh! You are so young. Give yourself time and you will conceive. Why go to a fertility clinic now?'

These 'free-ka-advice'-giving people rarely know that there are conditions like tubal blockage, bad sperm quality, low anti-Müllerian hormone (AMH) reserve, fibroids, genetic issues, endometriosis and polycystic ovary syndrome (PCOS) that deteriorate and complicate with time.

In my case, I was able to conceive naturally, but the pregnancy never sustained beyond the first term. In cases like mine, since you can conceive naturally, couples usually stick around with their gynae longer. People tell you that as long as you are able to conceive naturally there is nothing to worry. There is always a next time. It was only after my second miscarriage that I began thinking about seeing a fertility doctor. Meanwhile, I was losing my self-esteem, mind and heart, fretting over a million reasons why the miscarriage had happened. Was it because I was working, because I wore heels or because I had eaten a pineapple?

It sounds silly but it's true. All those who have conceived normally get the bragging rights. Theories with absolutely no correlation to science or logic come floating from every direction. It was only after a few years of suffering mental and emotional harassment that I realized that not all advice is good advice. When you are emotionally weak, you tend to soak in more and feel stressed and guilty about it.

Conception is a complex process.

Once, a guy from Lucknow called me and told me that he and his wife hadn't been able to conceive for the past three years and they were in distress. I was impressed that he spoke to me quite freely and confidently about the issue because it's rather uncommon for men to be so candid about infertility.

'You should go to a fertility clinic. It is quite late already', I told him.

'Madamji, agar kissi ne humey IVF clinic ke bahar bhi dekh liya toh ghar pe bahut bada bawaal ho jayega. Koi aur tareeka bata dijiye [Madam, if anyone sees us outside an IVF clinic then there'll be major drama at home. Tell me another way out].'

I was surprised to find that although he could talk to me freely under anonymity, he froze when he realized that he had to take his problem to a public setting. Ah! Social mindset. We can't change society, but we can change ourselves, right? One step at a time will surely transform the social behaviour towards fertility health soon.

Then there are people who run to babas and ojhas, waste more time, cause irreversible harm to their mind and body, and often escalate a simple problem to a chronic issue. Think about it like this. If you come down with dengue, you go see a doctor immediately, so why ponder a hundred times about seeing a fertility doctor if you're having trouble conceiving?

It's Time to Let Go of Your Gynaecologist

Shveta Suri, thirty-eight years, resident of Gurugram, tells me this:

We started trying for a baby only when I turned thirty. So, we tried for some time, and there was no luck. After one year of trying and no success I went to my GP, which in the United Kingdom (UK) is your general practitioner, the doctors that we go to. I told my GP that we have been trying and I am over thirty, so what to do? She did not see the situation as very serious; she just said that I'm being nervous and stressed out. I should relax. She did not do any scans or tests, and only verbally gave us this advice. She said it's no problem and it's the early side of thirties, so there should not be much problem. I should just keep trying. A few more months went by and there was still no success, so I changed my GP, and the new GP ran some tests. It was then that they diagnosed some issues and concluded that I may need assistance in conception. It took three years.[8]

Some (I am not saying all) gynaecologists will hold you longer than they should, and you need to be conscious of this. Again, some gynaecologists these days claim to be infertility/IVF experts for marketing purpose but in truth they don't have the requisite equipment (such as an embryology lab, intrauterine insemination [IUI]/IVF setup, etc.) or the degree or expertise, but rather have tie-ups with other IVF clinics to do procedures such as IUI or IVF or laproscopy or fibroid removal, as the case maybe. So basically, they will at some point in time refer you to an IVF clinic (if required) and take

---

8   Interview with Shveta Suri, thirty-three years old, Gurugram.

a small commission for providing a patient to the clinic (this is not an ethical practice and not everyone follows it). In all this, you end up wasting crucial time and patience. However, as much as it sounds good to be in the comfort zone (simply going to a gynae), you need to act quickly.

The other option is to consult a fertility specialist without leaving the trusted gynaecologists in the early stages. Compare the notes from both and make an informed decision.

When I asked Jaisnavi (thirty-two years old, working in the information technology [IT] sector) from Hyderabad how and when she left her gynaecologist to consult a fertility specialist, she said:

> I got married in July 2010. We were trying for a child since April 2011. For six to eight months, I consulted a gynaecologist. At that point, I was working in Hyderabad. Somebody told me about a gynaecologist who was close to my house and I went to her for six months. She kept me on ovulation medicine but nothing happened. In late 2012 to early 2013, I consulted an infertility specialist at Artemis. Since nothing else was working out, and we had already tried treatments and other medicines with the gynaecologist, we felt that we needed to see a fertility expert for specialized treatment. We were also a bit desperate by then.[9]

---

9   Interview with Jaisnavi, thirty-two years old, IT professional, Hyderabad.

Early Symptoms of Fertility Issues

Did you know that there are some glaring symptoms and signs of infertility that you can rectify even before you decide to start a family?

The problem with most couples is that they don't deal with these symptoms earlier; rather they wait until infertility hits them hard. Most people think that when they want kids all they need to do is have unprotected, timed sex and soon after they will be cradling a smiling baby in their arms. This happens for some people. But it need not work out so well for others.

The key to dodge escalation of fertility issues is to be prepared about it. Know the signs and take preventive steps. Many infertility cases are triggered by lifestyle issues. Here are a few things you need to be aware of:

Keep a Close Watch on Periods

This is perhaps the best and first indicator of infertility in women. Anything unusual—heavy, light, irregular/no periods at all, brown spotting prior to onset, extremely painful (not to be confused with regular cramps that are painful as well) are all symptoms that something's fishy. Periods are connected very closely to ovulation, and any irregularity or absence of ovulation only complicates your chances of getting pregnant.

Box 1.1: Best Sex Position for Getting Pregnant

> Sex positions that allow for deep penetration are better as they allow the sperm to be deposited as close to the cervix as possible. The good old 'missionary position' or the 'male partner on top' is often recommended for this reason. For additional support, after having sex, the woman can place a pillow under the hips to tilt the pelvis and help the sperm to 'travel'.

Source: Created by the author.

Hair Loss/Growth of Hair in Unusual Places and Acne

All of these are glaring symptoms of PCOS. Hair loss or acne could be the result of an auto-immune disease or thyroid malfunction, too, but they are usually the biggest symptoms of PCOS, so don't neglect it. Similarly, if you notice unusual facial and body hair growth, it is an indication of over-production of androgens, which is another clear indicator of PCOS. You must visit your doctor so that you can start medication immediately. One in every six women in India goes through PCOS, which often escalates into a fertility problem at a later stage. PCOS is the most common female endocrine disorder with a highly variable prevalence estimate, ranging from 2.2 to 26 per cent. The manifestations of PCOS may develop in adolescence but may not be diagnosed until well into adulthood. It is believed that both genetic predisposition and lifestyle factors contribute to the etiology of PCOS. Identifying and treating adolescents with PCOS is of prime importance, as adult women with PCOS have a tenfold increased risk of developing Type 2 diabetes, and a twofold increased risk of the metabolic syndrome.[10]

We will be discussing more about PCOS infertility in the following chapters.

Overweight/Underweight

Some women might notice that without any significant alterations in their diet or lifestyle, they gain or lose weight beyond healthy limits. This is an alarming situation. It is commonly seen that overweight/underweight women also suffer from menstrual dysfunction. However, being excessively under or overweight to what extent increases a woman's risk for infertility is unknown.[11]

These could be signs of fluctuations in the thyroid level or PCOS as well and must be addressed immediately.

---

10 R. Nidhi, V. Padmalatha, R. Nagarathna and R. Amritanshu, 'Prevalence of Polycystic Ovarian Syndrome in Indian Adolescents', *Journal of Pediatric and Adolescent Gynecology* 24, no. 4 (2011), pp. 223–27.

11 B.B. Green, N.S. Weiss and J.R. Daling, 'Risk of Ovulatory Infertility in Relation to Body Weight', Fertility and Sterility 50, no. 5(1988): 721–26.

Poor Gut Health or Digestive System

Gut health plays an important role in fertility. If you have frequent irritable bowel syndrome (IBS), bloating and discomfort, leaky bowel syndrome, gut dysbiosis, all these could be early warning signs. Esterobolome, the gut bacterial genes, play an important role in metabolizing estrogen. If this is not brought under control, it increases estrogen levels in the gut, which might be responsible for infertility later.

Premature Ageing

If you are in your thirties but experience signs of biological ageing like sagging breasts, dryness in the vagina, hair loss, brittle nails, these could be the first warning signs of infertility. These might (not definitely) mean that the quality and quantity of your eggs is decreasing. You need to visit a reproductive endocrinologist and get your hormones checked.

There are some tests like AMH, thyroid stimulating hormone (TSH), follicle stimulating hormone (FSH), haemoglobin (HB), thyroid, to name a few, that you must undergo at the early stages of planning a pregnancy. These tests are generally suggested when you are approaching IVF. I would say that there is no harm in getting the tests done early to be doubly sure. You must speak to your doctor about this. I shall discuss in detail the tests and diagnosis process in Chapter 2.

Decreased Sex Drive (in Both Men and Women)

Stress or depression causes decreased sex drive. There is no harm in meeting a psychologist to talk it out. While a little stress is normal, chronic or severe stress can be harmful. Alternatively, you can also take a vacation!

In some women, PCOS or endometriosis can reduce sexual drive and make having regular intercourse extremely painful. Among men, changes in virility could mean hormonal fluctuations, too, and therefore might be linked to infertility.

Testicle Pain or Small, Firm Testicles

Pain or swelling in the testicles could be attributed to many factors, but one of them could be infertility. Moreover, since testicles house the sperm, small or firm testicles can indicate issues that might make it difficult to impregnate.

Problems with Erection/Ejaculation

Erectile dysfunction or the inability to ejaculate is linked to hormonal imbalance. Therefore, it needs medical intervention early on. Azoospermia is another male infertility problem which is on the rise these days. Forty per cent of infertility cases are attributed to male reasons. Investigate further if you experience early signs of erectile dysfunction.[12]

---

12 N. Kumar and A.K. Singh, 'Trends of Male Infertility, an Important Cause of Infertility: A Review of Literature', Journal of Human

Box 1.2: Lying Down After Intercourse

> Many women ask if lying down after the intercourse would be ideal and for how long? Again, there is no research that backs this, but 10–15 minutes of lying down flat would be fine and anything longer is absolutely unnecessary. This will specially help if the semen gets ejaculated immediately from the vagina, after sex or in cases of lower sperm motility. Use this idle time to talk with your partner and build positive bonding.

Source: Created by the author.

Infertility doesn't happen overnight. Being conscious and proactive can save a lot of time and unnecessary stress at a later stage.

Box 1.3: Takeaway Points

> 1. Acknowledge that the problem exists.
> 2. Let go of any social taboos and go see a fertility doctor.
> 3. Don't listen to random advice.
> 4. Don't feel alone or guilty.
> 5. Don't delay diagnosis. Begin preparation early.
> 6. Don't panic and be gentle on yourself.

Source: Created by the author.

Reproductive Sciences 8, no. 4 (2015), pp. 191–96, available at https://www.ncbi.nlm.nih.gov/pmc/articles/PMC4691969/.

Being proactive is the best you can do. Fertility issues crop up because of lifestyle disorders. This gives us hope because lifestyle can be corrected and modified with right information and a bit of will power. Fertility issues build up gradually over time, and therefore, to reverse it will also take time. It won't happen overnight or magically. You must be patient and trust the journey, even though it comes unplanned and takes you through a discombobulate journey testing your mind and body at every pit stop.

2
Tests, Tests and More Tests

THERE IS A MEDICAL CONDITION CALLED 'UNEXPLAINED infertility' where doctors do all the tests but can't say for sure what is wrong and so they can't, in a concrete way, move forward towards a solution. I was a case of unexplained infertility and so are 10 per cent of all infertility cases, as per statistics. These are the worst because they keep doing tests and everything comes out normal, and still they are not getting pregnant. So, there is a point where you actually pray that some test report does come wrong so that then for sure you know what is wrong.

Unexplained infertility is like throwing darts in the dark.

Year after year, for ten years, I underwent all the tests that are out there—from vaginal scans to laparoscopy, hysterosalpingography (HSG)—injections were poked into every possible body part. Lie down, open your legs, stay calm, bear the pain, and then repeat. I felt naked, stripped of my dignity, and still there was no conclusive diagnosis.

During one of the tests, I was given a hospital robe, and post phase 1 of the test, the nurse nonchalantly asked me to go to another room for the next phase. I was in such distress that I didn't realize my robe was loosely tied at the back. My husband, Soumen, came rushing in to hold the robe, at which moment I had already passed many a people in the gallery. We walked like that, clutching each other, till the end of the gallery. That night, I held my hubby tightly and said, 'I feel so naked.' We both cried like babies.

The Horror of the HSG Test

I can never forget that evening when the doctor said, 'Get your HSG test done first and then we will see what we can do in your case.'

I followed the junior doctor like a sheep while Soumen was asked to make the payment. I was taken to what looked like a mini operation theatre (OT), given a blue gown to put on and asked to lie down on the surgical table. Overwhelmed by the complete setup, I sheepishly asked, 'Will it hurt?'

'Look ma'am', the junior doctor said, 'We will insert a dye in your uterus, and it will travel all through the uterus and fallopian tubes while we will take some scans of the uterus to determine if there is a blockage apart from some other analysis. You will feel a little discomfort.'

I was sceptical. I knew that pain was inevitable, but I wasn't prepared for the intensity of it.

Soon, I was writhing in excruciating pain and screaming. I had never ever experienced such physical pain before. It seemed to tear my internal organs apart. Instead of showing compassion, the junior doctor vociferously opinionated on how I was unfit to become a mother if I couldn't even bear this pain calmly.

The Necessary Evil Phase

Tests are the necessary evil phase. There are so many tests involved in this process that distress, discomfort and anxiety are natural.

The bigger problem is not the tests themselves but 'not understanding what these tests are for'.

Anxiety becomes a standard state of mind as we don't know why a particular test is important, what will it lead to, what to expect out of it and the process of the test. Mostly, you keep going for tests after tests because your doctor has said so.

On an average, a woman has to go through fifty to seventy tests during her fertility treatment. These tests are uncomfortable, quite frequent, inconclusive, and usually expensive.

When I asked Hanshika, a resident of Mumbai, about her experience of the diagnostic stage, she recalls:

> I think in a month I had to go through some 12 to 15 tests, varying from blood tests to ultrasounds.

I would've gone through some 40 to 45 tests in total during each cycle. All the tests were definitely uncomfortable. I used to feel very bothered while going for them.[13]

The Doctor's Perspective

Now there are two sides to this story—the patient and the doctor. Let us explore the doctor's side as it is important to set the right perspective and expectations.

Doctors follow a process of negation during fertility diagnosis, which simply means that they will rule out 'what is *not* wrong with you' to reach to a point where they hope to identify the reason of infertility. There are chances that there might be multiple culprits in your case. Infertility is a complex problem. The reasons for infertility can lie with the female or male or a combination of both the partners. Therefore, a couple has to go through so many tests before any conclusive diagnosis can be reached.

However, the problem with doctors is lack of communication. That's why I am writing this book—to bridge the communication gap for the sake of improved fertility treatment management by the patients themselves.

Doctors are busy, and though they understand the anxieties and empathize with the patient, they might not have enough time to deal with all your questions.

The trick to managing your restlessness is to *know*.

---

13   Author's interview with Hanshika, a Mumbai resident.

Finding A Fertility Doctor at the Initial Stage

When it is just six months to one year of not being able to conceive naturally and you are starting to think there might be a problem in conceiving. Or wondering why it is not happening naturally. At this initial stage, it is important to go to a fertility doctor who can get the process started. This fertility doctor can be from a clinic closest to your home or office or a recommendation of a friend/trusted online website. At this stage, deep research of the doctor is not required. That comes into play only when you have to go for any Assisted Reproductive Technology (ART) procedures like IUI or IVF. We will cover all aspects of choosing the right IVF doctor in Chapter 6.

Checklist of the Most Common Fertility Tests

Here is a list of tests that are commonly done during the fertility diagnosis phase.[14] It is important to prepare well for the test and keep calm as some of the tests are hormone-driven. Factors like anxiety or stress can adversely impact the test results. Doctors will then ask you to go for a re-test in the next month to confirm the results.

---

14   This is not a fully inclusive list as doctors might advise special tests based on your particular condition. However, these are some of the most common tests.

1. Comprehensive Blood Test

This is mainly to check for HB or blood-related infections. This is the most basic and common test that you will be advised when planning a pregnancy.

- Ideal HB levels in women trying to conceive should be within 12–15 g/dl. If your HB levels aren't in the correct range, don't worry, as this is the easiest of parameters to manage. HB levels increase by taking iron tablets and by following a proper diet.
- White Blood Cell (WBC) count should be between 4,000 and 10,000/uL.

Level—Basic | **Discomfort**—Low

2. Luteinizing Hormone (LH) Test

The LH is responsible for triggering ovulation. The test diagnoses if your eggs are ovulating in the way they should or should not be.

The FSH and LH tests are used in combination to help confirm the diagnosis of PCOS. Ideally, the FSH level should be higher than the LH level. The ratio of LH to FSH, when measured in international units, is elevated in women with PCOS. Common cut-offs to designate abnormally high LH/FSH ratios are 2:1 or 3:1, as tested on Day 2 or 3 of the menstrual cycle.

Very low levels of FSH and LH may indicate hypogonadotropic hypogonadism (HH).[15] High levels of FSH and LH may indicate impending or established menopause.

Level—Basic | **Discomfort**—Low

3. FSH Test

FSH stimulates the growth of ovarian follicles to prepare them for ovulation. This test has to be done on the second or third day of the period.

FSH levels over 10 mIU/ml indicates diminished fertility, poor egg health or a low ovarian reserve. The ovarian reserve may be low even in the presence of normal FSH levels. Due to this, other tests such as the AMH and the Antral Follicle Count on ultrasound are now preferred to assess your ovarian reserve.

Level—Basic | **Discomfort**—Low

4. AMH Test

This test tells you about your ovarian reserve. A woman is born with a certain number of eggs. So, if the AMH count

---

15 It means that there will be issues with ovaries and periods (less or no periods); there might also be low sex drive and an increase of male-like symptoms like body hair, etc.

is less it means that the ovarian reserve is fast depleting and that her biological clock is ticking faster.

Table 2.1: AMH Counts and What They Mean

Low	<0.3 ng/ml (Indicates diminished ovarian reserve)
Borderline Low	0.3–0.7 ng/ml
High	0.7–3.5 ng/ml
Borderline High	3.5–5.0 ng/ml
High	>5.0 ng/ml (Indicates PCOS)

Source: Created by the author.

Level—Intermediate | **Discomfort**—Low

5. Progesterone Hormone Test

The primary function of the hormone, progesterone, is to stimulate the growth of the uterus lining that helps the embryo to stick, settle and grow. This is the reason progesterone shots are given during the first trimester post-IVF conception.

Level—Intermediate | **Discomfort**—Moderate

6. Prolactin Hormone

The hormone, prolactin, is associated with milk production in pregnant and lactating woman. One of the causes of infertility in women is when prolactin count is high, which causes problems with ovulation. This is conducted through a blood test.

Prolactin level over 25 ng/ml indicates hyperprolactinemia (high prolactin condition) and may require treatment to bring it down before proceeding with IVF treatment.

Level—Intermediate | **Discomfort**—Low

7. Oestradiol or Estradiol

Remember, this blood test is done on the second or third day of your period. This test ascertains if your reproductive cycle is working well and is in sync with your ovulation cycles and patterns.

Oestradiol is one of the four types of oestrogen that the ovary produces. Oestradiol levels can affect how the reproductive system develops. Abnormal levels of oestradiol can cause menstrual problems, infertility, ovarian tumours or breast cancer.

Ideally, the levels should be less than 80 pg/ml on day two or three of the cycle. Elevated levels along with high FSH might indicate poor ovarian reserve. Again, certain cysts in the ovaries are known to produce oestrogen, and the levels would be high if the cysts are hormonally active. Very low oestrogen along with high FSH indicates a near-menopausal status, indicating very poor ovarian reserve.

Level—Basic | **Discomfort**—Low

8. TSH

This hormone regulates many bodily functions, including reproduction, and any imbalance in its levels has a direct effect on ovulation.

- Normal range is 0.27–4.20 mU/ml.
- In women who are trying to get pregnant, it is preferable to keep the level at or below 2.50 mU/ml. This is ideal for conception.

Level—Basic | **Discomfort**—Low

9. Antibody Test

In women who experience recurrent miscarriages, it is usually believed that they have a condition wherein the antibodies in their system have a tendency to fight their own foetus. This test is done to rule out such a condition.

Level—Intermediate | **Discomfort**—Low

10. HSG

This is the *baap* of all diagnostic tests. The HSG is an X-ray that checks the fallopian tubes to rule out blockage. It is usually done under sedation everywhere else in the world but not in India (I have no idea why), and this is the most painful of all tests. A medical dye is injected inside your uterus and is made to pass through the tubes to ensure that they are not blocked. This test is primarily conducted to check for tubal blockage, shape and overall working of the uterus.

When Mona, who was undergoing fertility treatments, was asked which is that one test you remember distinctively during the diagnosis phase, pat came the reply: 'HSG is the one I remember distinctly because it was about pushing some dye into the uterus and seeing the fluid spill out of me. So that to me was very scary because I experienced a lot of pain. Yeah, that is one that I remember very distinctly.'[16]

Level—Advanced | **Discomfort**—High

11. Laparoscopy

This is an advanced test because it requires a minor surgery in the abdomen and is performed under general anaesthesia. Small incisions are made, and the surgery is performed using laser technique. A camera is inserted while injecting huge amount of CO_2 gas into the abdomen, which often causes nausea, bloating and a heavy feeling once the patient comes out of anaesthesia. Detailed investigations of all reproductive organs are carried out. If minor endometriosis or cysts are found during the procedure, they are removed using laser while the procedure is on. You must rest after this procedure.

---

16 Author's interview with Mona.

This test is advised for those who might have endometriosis or fibroid issue.

Level—Advanced | **Discomfort**—High

12. Follicular Cycle Study

In this test, you are asked to do an ultrasound almost every alternate day during your ovulation period. The study primarily checks the cycle of egg formation, numbers formed, and whether the eggs are rupturing on time and properly. This is an important test and is especially done as a workup to IVF. Information from this test comes in handy for egg retrieval. The IVF process is done in two parts: first, egg retrieval is a surgical process done under anaesthesia, and second, after a few days the embryo transfer is carried out.

Level—Advanced | **Discomfort**—Moderate

13. Tuberculin Skin Test

This test is quite common, especially in India, and in cases of unexplained infertility. It is believed that underlying or latent tuberculosis can be a reason for not being able to conceive, IVF failure or recurrent miscarriages. In a test, a fluid is injected into the lower part of your arm, a circle is marked around that injection area, and then you are asked to come back after forty-eight to seventy-two hours to assess the test report.

During this time, a small lump will form where the injection has been administered. You might feel itchy and a slight discomfort.

Doctors will then see the lump physically and measure it, if required, to determine whether you have indications of tuberculosis or not. As this is not a conclusive test, if the doctor feels that there is some chance of tuberculosis, then they will ask for more follow up tests like a repeat of this skin test or a biopsy.

A lump size of more than 5 mm is considered positive.

Level—Advanced | **Discomfort**—High

14. Random Blood Sugar (RBS) Test

With India being the diabetes capital of the world,[17] we can't ignore the impact of diabetes on pregnancy. Your levels are considered normal if the count is between 80 and 160 mg/dl. However, anything above this is not good. If you are pre-diabetic, or have a history of diabetes in your family, it is better to take precautionary steps both in terms of medical treatment and holistic lifestyle management to prevent it from escalating at a later stage.

---

17   S.K. Pandey and V. Sharma, 'World Diabetes Day 2018: Battling the Emerging Epidemic of Diabetic Retinopathy', Indian Journal of Ophthalmology 66, no. 11 (2018), pp. 1652–53, available at https://pubmed.ncbi.nlm.nih.gov/30355895/.

Table 2.2: RBS Levels

Normal	80–160 mg/dl
Pre-diabetic	160–200 mg/dl
Diabetic range	>200 mg/dl

Source: Created by the author.

Level—Basic | **Discomfort**—Moderate

15. Vitamin D

Vitamin D has a direct effect on AMH production, and this increases the longevity of ovarian reserve in patients who have a higher concentration of it. So, don't take Vitamin D lightly. If it is low, which it is in most of the Indian population,[18] especially those working in offices and closed spaces, then you must take corrective measures.

Level—Basic | **Discomfort**—Low

16. Endometrial Receptivity Analysis (ERA)

ERA is a genetic test which analyses genes and evaluates the perfect time window when one's endometrial lining is ready to accept an embryo. Using latest technology, this

---

18 S. Ray, 'Indians are Vitamin D Deficient. And No, it Can't be Fixed by Diet Alone', *The Print*, 10 December 2021, available at https://theprint.in/opinion/indians-are-vitamin-d-deficient-and-no-it-cant-be-fixed-by-diet-alone/779535/.

advanced test assesses approximately 236 genes to predict the accurate time to place an embryo in the uterus for facilitating successful implantation leading to pregnancy. It has been found that in 25 per cent of IVF failure cases, the cardinal reason is displaced 'window of implantation', and ERA can plug this lack of clarity.

ERA is recommended for:

1. Women with two or more unsuccessful embryo transfers, that is, recurrent implantation failure.
2. Women with concerns regarding endometrial lining, like thin endometrial lining.
3. Women with unsuccessful implantation despite high-quality embryos.
4. Unexplained and multiple implantation failure.

ERA is a biopsy test of the endometrium lining. This test measures the 'receptive profile' of the endometrium for five days, after starting progesterone support. The patient will have to take hormone replacement therapy (HRT) medication (oestrogen and progesterone) till the ERA test biopsy day, which is day five, when the embryo transfer usually takes place. It's the time when the endometrial tissue primes itself for implantation. This tissue is carefully scrapped and investigated.

ERA is done during an IVF cycle to provide improved insights for the next cycle. The biggest drawback with an ERA test is that it can't help immediately. However, ERA makes logical sense in frozen IVF cycles where you only undergo embryo transfer.

For an in-depth discussion on types of IVF, see Chapter 7.

Harshita, thirty-two-year-old teacher staying in Delhi and trying to conceive past five years, says:

> The process was quite simple; it got over in just 10 minutes. There was only a tickling sensation with no pain throughout the process. But I felt some cramping, as we feel during periods, for two days post ERA treatment. However, the cramps were not severe and I was able to bear the same without much problem.[19]

Level—Advanced | **Discomfort**—Moderate

17. Preimplantation Genetic Screening (PGS)

PGS is an advanced genetic study of the embryos produced during the IVF cycle. This test screens the embryos for any kind of chromosomal abnormalities before transferring them into the uterus. PGS helps in improved embryo selection by determining the chromosome number of each embryo growing into the blastocyst stage. One of the reasons for implantation failure is genetically abnormal embryos that look perfectly good from the outside but

---

19 Author's interview with Harshita, thirty-two-year-old Delhi resident.

won't implant; and even if they do implant, it will lead to early miscarriage. Thus, PGS is recommended to eliminate this from occurring.

PGS works along with the IVF cycle. Once the embryos are made, a sample of each is sent for genetic assessment. Based on the reports, only embryos marked chromosomally correct are transferred into the uterus during the embryo transfer stage.

PGS is recommended in the following cases:

1. **Advanced maternal age:** Generally, chromosomal abnormalities increase with increase in the age of women. So, women over thirty-five years are recommended PGS to avoid later complications.
2. **Recurrent failures:** More than half of early miscarriages and implantation failure are attributed to chromosomal abnormalities. PGS is recommended in cases of multiple IVF failure and recurrent miscarriages.
3. **Precious embryo:** If in your case only one good embryo was formed, and the doctor decides to transfer a single embryo, then you can increase chances of your implantation success by getting the PGS test, which will ensure that the embryo does not have any deformity or genetic issues. It is a simple math of probability where you increase your success chances, though nothing can be guaranteed. If you already have low AMH and are making limited numbers of follicles, then it is best to put all your efforts into making the IVF cycle successful.

4. **Severe male factors:** Embryos formed with severe male infertility issues like deoxyribonucleic acid (DNA) fragmentation of sperm or higher DNA fragmentation index (DFI) might have issues in implantation, thereby leading to miscarriage or having a genetic issue of parents transferred to the baby. Thus, PGS screening simply minimizes the risks and increases the probability of success. PGS helps to rule out the incompatible embryos.

Level—Advanced | **Discomfort**—Low (as this test is done in the laboratory and not on you.)

Male Infertility Tests

Did you know that 40 per cent of infertility is due to male fertility issues? Doctors usually advise the basic sperm test in the first one or two consultations. It is logical to assess basic male fertility parameters before moving on to higher level investigations. However, owing to social conditioning, sometimes men go into denial mode, and it defeats the path of recovery.

1. Semen Analysis

This test ascertains the quality of semen based on volume, count, motility and morphology. This is a basic test and usually the beginning point of fertility testing for men. However, there are few other tests like hormone tests and testicular biopsy, which might be advised based on your individual medical case.

The normal range for sperm count is 40–300 million sperm/ml

Remember to abstain from sex or masturbation twenty-four hours before the test.

There are several other tests to check fertility in men, but fortunately (for men) in India they are not so popular.

Level—Basic | **Discomfort**—Low

2. DFI

Baby-making is nothing but passing your genes to the embryo, and thus, having your 'biological child'. However, if there is some problem in the genes or DNA of the male, it leads to higher DFI of the sperm, which might lead to unhealthy embryos. Such embryos would either not get implanted, leading to delayed pregnancy, or if implanted might lead to early miscarriage or passing of bad DNA in the child causing complications at a later stage.

DFI is an advanced test for men to rule out any genetic issue. Higher DFI is indicative of DNA damage of the sperm. Please note that higher DFI only means that a higher percentage of sperms might have gene damage. If your DFI is higher, don't worry too much and remember that all you need is one sperm to make the embryo.

Cases of unexplained infertility, recurrent miscarriages, recurrent IVF failures and abnormal sperm report are recommended to get this test done, based on which further line of fertility treatment is advised.

Level—Advanced | **Discomfort**—Low

Fertility Test for the Couple

Interestingly, infertility is the only medical problem where two people get treated simultaneously. Understandably, this makes it all the more difficult to diagnose the root cause. Both men and women are advised to undergo multiple tests to identify the cause of infertility. However, in cases of advanced stages of infertility and mostly unexplained infertility, couple tests are suggested.

Genetic Counselling

When none of the above tests provide a conclusive diagnosis and the reason of infertility remains a mystery, then fertility specialists turn to genetic counselling. This is expensive and starts with a chromosome profile test where chromosomes are checked for any structural or profiling anomaly. Genetic testing is done for both the partners. If you had a miscarriage and/or a planned/surgical abortion, also called dilation and curettage (D&C), was performed, then the remnants of the embryo are also sent for genetic testing to find a conclusive answer to why the miscarriage happened so that the course of the fertility treatment can be corrected, and the couple is able to conceive soon.

When I had my third miscarriage, D&C was done to remove the embryo and it was sent for genetic testing. The report didn't help much in understanding the cause of miscarriage or infertility, but it did say that it was a male embryo, and for many nights I would dream of a baby boy going away from me. I wish I didn't know it was a male embryo as it became all the more difficult to overcome the grief of miscarriage. It now had a face.

Level—Advanced | **Discomfort**—Low

Box 2.1: Pro Tip

> **Overall, you need to be mindful of the following aspects:**
>
> 1. Are your periods regular?
> 2. Have you noticed excess weight gain recently?
> 3. Have you developed excessive facial hair recently?
>
> Make a note of any such changes and speak to your doctor.

Source: Created by the author.

Psychological and Lifestyle Tests

Did you know that in earlier times a couple had to pass psychological screening or you can call it an emotional preparedness test before being allowed to go for IVF? Such is the importance of psychological well-being which we sadly ignore in modern times.

While medical diagnostic tests are important and most stressed upon, psychological and lifestyle tests are often completely ignored. These are the slow-killing factors which play a key role in impacting fertility. Age, nutrition, psychological stress, anxiety, irregular sleep cycle, lack of exercise, smoking or drinking habits, occupational exposures, disturbed relationships, and even caffeine consumption can adversely impact fertility.

The good thing about psychological and lifestyle-related issues is that *they are under your control*. You can assess, modify and control them with a positive impact being visible almost immediately.

Below are some of the factors that you have to self-assess and self-manage to get positive results in minimum time.

1. Age

Age plays a critical role in your reproductive timeline. However much our parents or grandparents crib, coax and cajole us to marry and have kids early, the truth is that in the twenty-first century, higher education, and career and settlement graphs have pushed marriage and childbearing to much later. In urban areas, people are only getting married at around twenty-eight to thirty years.[20] Then post a year of mandatory honeymoon period begins the journey towards the next phase, that is, parenthood. By this time, they are in their early thirties. Whereas the ideal age of conception is below thirty-five.

S. Ganguly and S. Unisa identify the trends of infertility and childlessness in India thus:

> Census of 1981 estimates infertility in India around 4-6 percent and according to NFHS-1 childlessness is around 2.4 percent of currently married women over 40 years in India (cited in Jejeebhoy, 1998). Childlessness in India is estimated around 2.5 percent. It is around 5.5 percent for 30-49 age group and 5.2 percent for 45-49 age group. In absolute terms it is around 4.9 million and if secondary infertility is also added to it then the total number of infertile couples is around 17.9 million.[21]

---

20 Hans News Service, 'Late Marriages Pushing Couples into Infertility, Expert Says', *The Hans India*, 10 November 2021, available at https://www.thehansindia.com/karnataka/late-marriages-pushing-couples-into-infertility-says-expert-714568.

21 S, Unisa and S. Ganguly, 'Trends of Infertility and Childlessness in India: Findings from NFHS Data', *Facts, Views and Vision in Obstetrics and Gynaecology* 2, no. 2 (2010), pp. 131–38, available at https://www.ncbi.nlm.nih.gov/pmc/articles/PMC4188020/.

Even though the reproductive potential of women declines post thirty-five years, we are taking much better care of ourselves in terms of awareness about nutrition and exercise. This means that we might be able to manage the biological clock a little bit. The correlation between age and fertility is associated with our eggs. Women are born with a certain number of eggs, and with each cycle of ovulation they waste a few eggs. Women peak, in terms of fertility, around their twenties and then the gradual decline begins from thirties till the forties. Though they might be ovulating in their forties, one can't be sure about the quality of eggs. In fact, 'there is a sharp decline in fertility in women post 35 years of age.'[22]

On the other hand, there have been cases in which young women have been diagnosed with declining egg/ovarian reserve. And, then there are women who conceive perfectly at a so-called older age.

So, even though generally age and biological clock tick together, it also depends on the individual. The only sure shot way of assessing and staying ahead of your biological clock is to get periodic tests done, namely AMH. This will clearly tell where you stand in terms of your ovarian reserve—basically the available age window that you have to plan your family so that you can take a scientifically backed, informed decision. This is powerful information for both unmarried women who would currently like to focus on

---

[22] J. Menken, J. Trussell and U. Larsen, 'Age and infertility' *Science* 233, no. 4771(1986), pp. 1389–94, available at https://www.science.org/doi/10.1126/science.3755843.

their career and for married women who wish to postpone childbearing to a later date without any risk or regret.

For others, the golden window to have children is below thirty-five years and ideally between twenty-seven and thirty-two years. So, plan and stick to this window.

What if I miss the window?

Well, medical science has progressed so much that there is always a way. You just need to know and take action in advance.

Egg freezing is your answer.

The process of egg freezing is pretty much the same as the initial phase of IVF. Initially, a fertility specialist will analyse your reproductive health and will recommend pills to bypass the menstrual cycle.

You will be given rounds of hormone injections to stimulate the ovaries for about one to two weeks. You will need to make regular visits to the fertility clinic to check the health of the ovaries. When the eggs are seen to be mature enough, they are retrieved by using a needle, inserted with the help of ultrasound, and stored safely.

You can easily freeze the eggs between seven and ten years.

Let's now focus our attention on men. In terms of fertility and age, they fare better than the fairer sex. Fertility in men begins to decline post forties. Their window is much broader comparatively.

2. Weight

Being overweight or underweight is not a good thing. You know that already, right? It is always indicative of an underlying or undiagnosed issue. Mostly in the case of fertility treatment, the issue is either PCOS or thyroid.

Women with a body mass index (BMI) of:

- Less than 20 have 18 per cent longer delay in conceiving.
- 25–29 have a 17 per cent longer delay.
- 30–34 have a 25 per cent longer delay.
- Above 35 have a 39 per cent longer delay.

The ideal BMI should range between 20 and 24.

It is important to self-assess your weight and BMI periodically and keep track of it. Anything unusual should not be ignored. There are many health and wellness apps to help you with this. A simple weighing machine is also good enough.

3. Nutrition

Nutrition plays an important role in maintaining a healthy mind and body, and even more so for reproductive health. But there is a vicious cycle that many women fall into when they begin IVF procedures.

It begins with their doctor asking them to lose weight to increase their chances of conception. As this is the only factor within their control, and the most visible one for them and their family members, they begin a war against fat. They become oblivious to the fact that there were other medical factors for not being able to conceive. They go into fad diets thinking that once the weight reduces everything will fall into place. The problem with fad diets (keto, intermittent fasting, etc.) is that though they will drastically reduce weight in a shorter period of time, that might not be sustainable and is usually a lopsided management, leading to other health issues like triggering a migraine or a drop in blood sugar. It is best to focus on holistic lifestyle changes towards a sustainable, healthy living.

Ramiya, a thirty-one-year-old from Mumbai who works in a leading corporate suffered from endometriosis and fibroid (the main reason for infertility) and was overweight by 5–7 kgs. She went chasing weight loss like there was no tomorrow. Fad diets (almost to the point of not eating), exercising for hours and hopping onto the weighing machine became her daily routine. This madness was supported by her family, and no one raised an alarm. Soon, she fainted, her glucose levels plummeted, and she was diagnosed with severe anaemia, which derailed her fertility treatment by a few months as she had to recover from this self-created issue. Fad diets might show results on the outside, but they will impact your immunity, the strength of your uterus and the health of your reproductive organs. You need to have a healthy body not only to conceive, but also to bear the baby for nine months and thereafter. Be mindful of your weight and how you lose or gain it.

The point I'm trying to make here is that there is no shortcut to conception. Take every advice with a pinch of salt and don't go for solutions that offer quick results.

4. Lifestyle parameters

There are many lifestyle parameters that affect fertility. These are:

- **Exercise:** Are you exercising at least twice a week? Take a walk or do some light yoga, or anything, just move your body.
- **Sleep Cycle**: Monitor your sleep cycle. All of us know that eight hours of sleep is important but what about sleep quality and deep sleep time. You can get a Garmin® watch or a similar watch or even a health app to monitor your sleep and assess your sleep cycle.
- **Smoking/Alcohol intake**: Social drinking and smoking occasionally is fine. However, anything beyond a moderate level needs to be controlled. And this goes for both the partners. Even men need to be vigilant about their smoking and alcohol consumption.
- **Caffeine**: Usually, corporate or high-stress jobs lead to an increased intake of coffee. There is no conclusive research to connect coffee consumption with declined fertility rates. However, caffeine intake affects one's overall metabolism. This, in turn, impacts ovulation, menstruation and hormones.

- **Occupational impact**: Did you know that infertility is highest among urban couples working in the IT sector?[23] Do you know why? Occupational hazards. Obesity, delayed marriages, longer sitting hours, bad food habits and unhealthy lifestyle impacts immunity. PCOS, other menstrual and gynaecological issues are common effects, often escalating to requiring fertility treatment. Again, there is no conclusive research connecting infertility and the IT sector in India.

Then there are people in the armed and defence services who have to undergo involuntary infertility as men are posted away from families for a long period of time. People engaged in industries that involve strong chemicals also pose a threat to fertility. Similarly, in villages, farmers closely working with pesticides might show symptoms of infertility.[24]

If you work in a similar field, then take a rain check and plan your pregnancy.

---

23 N. Purkayastha and H. Sharma, 'Prevalence and Potential Determinants of Primary Infertility in India: Evidence from Indian demographic Health Survey', *Clinical Epidemiology and Global Health* 9 (January 2021), pp. 162–70, available at https://cegh.net/article/S2213-3984(20)30190-1/fulltext.

24 R. Sharma, K.R. Biedenharn, J.M. Fedor and A. Agarwal, 'Lifestyle Factors and Reproductive Health: Taking Control of Your Fertility', *Reproductive Biology and Endocrinology* 11, no. 66 (July 2013), available at https://rbej.biomedcentral.com/articles/10.1186/1477-7827-11-66.

5. Relationship Status

Couples going through fertility treatment have to handle many issues like social stigma, the distress of the invasive treatment process, added financial burden, the anxiety of the unknown, losing control over the future, and all this, in turn, leads to stress that takes a toll on relationships.

Indian families are tightly knit with parents and close relatives having a say in important matters. It is usually a lonely road for any woman undergoing fertility treatment. The lack of control over circumstances can make her mistrust everyone and everything around her. This is not a conducive environment for successful fertility treatment. So, in this case, **STOP TESTING YOUR RELATIONSHIPS**. Blaming each other for the situation of infertility causes fights in a relationship. And if a relationship is troubled, then how do you expect to have good sex, and thereby, conception? It is like a vicious cycle—you don't get pregnant, you take stress, out of which you blame your partner or behave in such a way that causes more rifts, leading to bad sex under the clock based on your ovulation window, and then no conception.

6. Psychological Tests

Do you feel continued stress, anxiety or distress?

Do you think that your basic nature is changing?

Do you have mood swings, irritability and irrational behaviour, which are beyond your control, and then you feel guilty later?

If you've answered yes to any of the above questions, you must meet a psychologist or counsellor or join a support group.

Support group has been found to be an effective way to reduce stress during fertility treatment. A focus on teaching relaxation, breathing, self-help techniques and self-awareness in a group setting is known to decrease stress. According to this study, psychosocial interventions, with an emphasis on cognitive behavioural therapy, could be effective in reducing psychological distress and they are also associated with a significant increase in pregnancy rates. Thus, cognitive behavioural therapy could be an effective way to reduce distress and improve pregnancy rates.[25]

If going to a psychologist is another taboo for you, then look for apps or online consultations, such as Fertility Dost, YourDost, BetterLYF, which provide support at your convenience and with anonymity. The important thing here is to not ignore this aspect.

How to Navigate the Diagnosis Phase

It usually takes a few menstrual cycles to undergo all fertility tests. As some of these are hormonal tests, results may fluctuate, and so your doctor might ask you to repeat the tests. Tests are an integral part of the fertility journey. It is

---

[25] K.L. Rooney and A.D. Domar, 'The Impact of Stress on Fertility Treatment', *Current Opinion in Obstetrics and Gynaecology* 28, no. 3 (2016), pp. 198–201, available at https://www.ncbi.nlm.nih.gov/pmc/articles/PMC4188020/.

a ladder that you climb, with every next step seeming more daunting than the previous one. Here are a few points to help you through this phase:

5. **Clear thinking**: It is very important to keep your head clear and not make decisions based on emotions.
6. **Hyper assessment of test results**: Doing a test, waiting to know the results, and comprehending the impact of the results on your treatment path can generally lead to a lot of anxiety. However, having patience and listening to what the experts say, then taking one step at a time to resolve the issue is a much better approach. Often, couples spend a lot of time googling symptoms and tests, asking all the wrong people, getting too much unsolicited advice, and trying too hard to improve the test parameters. This is not the correct approach.

Fertility is a complex and layered issue. There can be multiple factors causing infertility; plus, diagnosis is based on assessing multiple factors and tests—both physical and diagnostic. You can't watch a YouTube video and start drinking fertility tea the whole day just because they are supposed to improve your fertility. This is a simplistic example to help you understand that you must keep that fine balance.

I see so many women every day getting unnecessarily stressed trying to work on their endometrium lining or to control weight, so much so that they let the stress impact the treatment itself.

7. **Stress-free environment**: It is easier said than done but it is not unachievable. Make sure to put a stopwatch on stress and anxiety you feel due to fertility issues. Make a vow to not let it linger on forever and take concrete steps to tackle it head on.
8. **Second opinion**: This will surely be a confusing time for you. You will feel unprepared to handle this situation. No Google search will ever answer all your questions. There are important decisions to be taken every day. Personally, I found the 'second opinion' technique quite useful. There is no harm in seeing two to three doctors for an opinion. They might push you to do some tests before they can delve further. So, be upfront and tell the doctor that you are here for a second opinion because you are either not fully convinced by the advice given by your current doctor or you want to get a particular aspect investigated further as you know your body better and have a gut feeling.

    Remember to do this without being condescending to the current doctor. This is so that the doctor you have gone to for the second opinion will have the right expectations and will give the best advice they can, for they know that if you end up liking their advice you might shift from your primary doctor. Compare their notes, dig deeper, and then make an informed choice. This is another way to research.
9. **Test report not satisfactory**: There might be a scenario when your heart says that the test reports on which

your current diagnosis is based is not correct. This can happen due to two reasons:

- **The test report really is wrong.** It happens all the time. Although as per the norms of the National Accreditation Board for Testing and Calibration Laboratories (NABL), all laboratories must be certified, some are franchises of big diagnostic brands and are not properly accredited. In these laboratories, because of lack of system and procedure, reports are often erroneous. Interpretation of test reports may vary from one doctor to another. Some might look at your AMH report and suggest an extreme line of treatment suggesting you plan for IVF immediately, while another doctor might interpret it as bad but not worse suggesting a moderate treatment path.

Box 2.2: What Should You Do?

- Follow your gut.
- Get the retest done from another lab.
- Look for a doctor who you think or know will work better for you.
- Take a second opinion.
- Compare notes of different doctors and see which doctor makes more sense.

Source: Created by the author.

- **You are too emotional to accept infertility** and that's why your heart is not being able to trust the tests and finding an excuse to delay the process of acceptance. Trust me, this happens more often than not.

What Should You Do?

Calm down. Never make a decision when you are too emotional. Give it some time. Let the emotions settle. Then think. Take the decision when you are more balanced and neutral. Take all the time you need but take the decision on further treatment plan when you are emotionally ready. So many couples hamper and derail their treatment because they are desperate for quick results. And you know that never works.

At this stage, a lot of folks also waste crucial time by running away from doctors and getting into a comfort zone like following Ayurveda, homoeopathy or some astrologer. If you hear stories about others who claim they got pregnant with the help of some *vaidji*, you should ask yourself: did they tell you every detail about their treatment? Is your fertility condition the same as theirs? Thus, will the same treatment plan work for you, too?

Alternative treatment methodologies should work in tandem with allopathic treatment. Just don't give up allopathic treatment especially if you are in the early stages of treatment. We will talk about late stages of infertility management in Chapter 12. This phase is about being introduced to the world of infertility, acceptance, about questioning social conditioning and adjusting your life goals.

Box 2.2: In Short...

> 1. Be informed before going for a test.
> 2. Know enough to get the test done properly but not too much since that would lead to anxiety. Thus, balance is key.
> 3. Anxiety and stress can give the wrong results as most of the tests are hormone-related. Stay calm.
> 4. Be patient during the test phase as fertility is not a simple issue where a bunch of tests lead to immediate diagnosis.
> 5. Be aware that the diagnosis phase might take time.

Source: Created by the author.

3
The Difficult Acceptance

'You never know how strong you are, until being strong is your only choice.'

— **Bob Marley**

INFERTILITY? WHAT RUBBISH!
I can't have infertility. I am young, healthy, and my periods come like clockwork. This doctor is surely mistaken, or, maybe, the test reports are flawed.

I came back home. My mother called me on the phone. She asked, 'What happened? What did the doctor say?'

'The doctor says that I might have infertility', I told her.

And then, without any warning, all hell broke loose.

'But you are conceiving, right? So how can it be infertility? Your uterus was weak and couldn't hold the baby, and that's why you had a miscarriage this time. It happens. You just need to try again and be very careful next time. You will have a baby soon.'

This love-laden scolding was so comforting that it reinforced my underlying thoughts that I couldn't possibly be infertile. Unfortunately, this mindset also delayed my acceptance of my condition. It took me almost two more years and two miscarriages to finally get me to wrap my head around the fact that I was, in fact, suffering from infertility. And so, I finally went back to the fertility consultant.

The Shock of Infertility

Being a parent is a cherished life goal for most people. No one questions whether they will become parents because it is a well-defined step in the timeline of life. After all, making a baby is a natural process, right? That's what we're all told and taught at school. We get married, and then when we want kids we will have unprotected sex, and the next thing we know is there will be a baby bump. Done!

When you are told that making a baby (a seemingly natural process) won't happen for you naturally, your social conditioning gets rocked to the core. At first, you are confused, after which you enter a vicious cycle of 'why' and 'how' it happened. Anxiety, fear, isolation, guilt, frustration and helplessness are just some of the initial emotions you are bound to go through. After all, you had a perfect plan—marriage, wait X number of years, then have the first baby, manage initial parenting challenges, then go back to work, and so on and so forth. For some of us, when all those plans fall apart, it begins to threaten our very identity.

The Difficult Acceptance

Infertility begins to feel like a huge failure of you as a woman or man (with whoever the major fault lies). You couldn't succeed at something as basic as conceiving, something that you should have had under your control. It seems like your life is going against societal norms. You get a sinking feeling. Being childless disqualifies a woman from being a member of the covetous 'mommy group'. You fear judgement, pity, and sarcastic remarks from friends and family, and society at large.

The reason we don't accept infertility as a simple medical issue, like, say, kidney stones, is because of our social conditioning. As per a study, a woman going through cancer and another going through infertility undergo similar physical and mental trauma.[26] However, a woman going through cancer is met with social empathy. People will say, 'Oh! Such a young girl and she got cancer,' whereas the woman going through infertility is met with social apathy. People around her will sarcastically remark, 'Oh! She focuses more on her job, is overweight, drinks and all; that is why she is not able to conceive. These young girls they don't even want to become mothers.'

---

26 A.D. Domar, P.C. Zuttermeister and R. Friedman, 'The Psychological Impact of Infertility: A Comparison with Patients with Other Medical Conditions, *Journal of Psychosomatic Obstetrics and Gynecology* 14 (1993): 45–52, available at https://pubmed.ncbi.nlm.nih.gov/8142988.

Anger, grief and conflict are the common emotions that you will experience. I felt these 'mood swings' uncontrollably and frequently during my fertility journey.

'I found out about my infertility after my first miscarriage. I was really depressed because that first miscarriage was heartbreaking,' says Fatima from Kolkata, a twenty-eight-year-old freelance graphic designer.

Depression is common and a significant part of couples experiencing infertility. Infertility-related stress and depression is higher in women because we tend to internalize the pain.[27] We blame ourselves mercilessly for infertility, and this guilt works as a catalyst to the fire of the pain within.

Couples undergoing infertility often feel anxious, isolated and a sense of losing control. It is natural to feel like this. Infertility is stressful and stress is not good for getting pregnant. So, what do you do? You learn and practise coping mechanisms because stopping is not an option …

> *'No matter how many times you get knocked down, keep getting back up. God sees your resolve. He sees your determination. And when you do everything you can do, that's when God will step in and do what you can't do.'*
>
> – **Joel Osteen**

---

[27] K.L. Rooney and A.D. Domar, 'The Relationship between Stress and Infertility', *Dialogues in Clinical Neuroscience* 20, no. 1 2018): 41–47, available at https://www.ncbi.nlm.nih.gov/pmc/articles/PMC6016043/.

Coping Strategies

1. Cope as a Couple, Not as Individuals

Different people cope differently when faced with stressful situations. How a couple copes with infertility plays a vital role in their fertility journey.

Coping strategies such as avoidance of the problem and accepting personal responsibility for one's infertility are commonly associated with increased distress, whereas coping strategies such as seeking social support and engaging in active problem-solving tend to decrease distress. The primary purpose of coping with infertility is to manage the emotional and/or behavioural reactions a couple experiences once a diagnosis of infertility is given. For example, couples will use coping strategies such as avoidance of the problem to deal with the unexpected news of infertility, their perceived loss of a child, or they may have difficulty in relating to friends with young children. Coping may also be used to reduce stress over infertility for the purpose of repairing rifts in the marital relationship or avoiding feelings of depression associated with multiple losses the couple perceives.[28]

---

28 B.D. Peterson, C.R. Newton, K.H. Rosen and R.S. Schulman, 'Coping Processes of Couples Experiencing Infertility', *Family Relations* 55, no. 2 (2006), 227–39, available at https://onlinelibrary.wiley.com/doi/abs/10.1111/j.1741-3729.2006.00372.x.

It is interesting to note that coping mechanisms for men and women in this scenario might be different, and often, this becomes the bone of contention between partners. Men and women think, react and behave differently—we all know that. Under this immensely stressful scenario, we tend to misunderstand each other, which leads to conflict in the relationship, thereby adding more stress. The result is usually a delay in treatment or wrong decisions taken under emotional distress. Many times, it feels like marriages are breaking down.

In my fertility journey, it felt like my marital relationship had hit rock bottom. I would often ask my husband to divorce me and marry someone else because I felt guilty, and my self-esteem was at its lowest. However, now, if he even looks at another woman, I will tear him apart.

That's the truth of life.

Marital adjustment is the key here. Men often cope by distracting themselves. They will throw themselves into work. Even if this seems inconsiderate, it doesn't mean that they care less. The wife, on the other hand, will drop everything and think about the fertility issue like a *tapasya*, vowing not to do anything else until she is blessed with a baby. She will stop going to parties, meeting people, and in most cases, even quit her job. I have come across many cases where women working in senior management positions have left their jobs to focus on their fertility treatment. Well, in this case, a small but vital part is also played by an apathetic corporate environment (more about balancing career and fertility treatment has been elaborated on in Chapter 9).

The Difficult Acceptance

Debashish (thirty-three) and his wife (thirty-one) lived in the US. He was in a senior position at his company and was going through her fertility journey. Debashish confided in me:

> Men don't have shoulders to cry on. Women have friends, mothers and sisters with whom they share, cry and at least vent out the feeling. In a man's case, owing to social conditioning, I can't talk about it with my friends over drinks. I am supposed to play the role of this strong and stoic man who has to take care of his wife as she is the one facing the bullet. I need to stand beside her and take the right decisions, do the right thing. But I am equally clueless about this whole journey. I am equally shocked and choked. Fertility is a new term for me too and dealing with it a new learning every day. Though I stand tall for the sake of my wife, but my heart is scared and cries all the time.[29]

This tells us a lot about how men feel and process the journey. So as a wife, you need to be mindful of your partner's emotions even though you are the one undergoing more physical and emotional distress.

Men find it difficult to distract themselves out of this messy issue. I call it 'messy' because fertility is an emotional rollercoaster and men find such scenarios uncomfortable.

---

29 Conversation with Debashish, a thirty-three-year-old, a US resident.

However, for the sake of your wife, to make the relationship work and to cope together, you must loudly and frequently tell your wife that you care, you understand, and you are with her.

Denial as a coping strategy is not good. If either of the partners is in denial, then it will push your partner away and cause unwarranted delay in the treatment path.

Sumita, resident of Durgapur, has been through sixteen years of fertility journey post which she conceived twins through IVF in her forties. She says:

> If your husband is supportive then managing infertility becomes a bit easier. For some people, the definition of a supportive husband is someone who provides food and money. For me, financial support is not that important. I need emotional support. But my husband does not give me any emotional support. Friends and family tell me that I am lucky to have such a good husband. When you meet him outside of the home, he is a very different person, very responsible. But when he comes home, he is like a feudal lord, a 1940s-type patriarchal male figure. He may be good and charming socially but at home he is that same patriarchal male chauvinist.
>
> The perfect groom is selected based on his looks, family background and earning potential. But is that the only thing? No. It is not. How you have been brought up and how you prioritize your relationship with your wife are important qualities. A

man must be able to emotionally segregate between his mother and wife to avoid typical mother-in-law and daughter-in-law relationship stress, especially when there is the added stress of infertility, an active volcano that is just waiting to explode.[30]

Women seek emotional support. They need constant reassurance that they are your priority. Most importantly, if your house also has the typical MIL versus DIL scenario, then cutting corners won't help. You need to find a solid solution. And you have to be proactive. It is difficult and will require extreme patience and diplomacy, but you've got to do what you've got to do.

The fertility journey is a mind game and having a strong partner can make a world of difference.

Control Extended Family Intervention

During your fertility journey, family support, love and care are indispensable. But the extended Indian family can be an obstacle to progress. In fact, often, our mothers or mothers-in-law won't be of much help as fertility is a new-age issue and they aren't aware about it holistically. Then, there are curious relatives who can't stop themselves from asking the *Kaun Banega Crorepati* question, 'So, when is the good news?', and you are expected to be all shy, coy and blushing. In fact, Bollywood has played its role in over-hyping this situation.

---

30 Interview with Sumita, a Durgapur resident.

Sunayna Uberoy, a twenty-seven-year-old teacher at an international school in Gurgaon, who is now also a proud mother of two daughters through adoption, says:

> The most difficult thing for me was meeting pregnant women. I would become jealous and hated them; so much so that I refused to work with them as well. Obviously, I did not want to go to any social event, baby showers, birthdays, etc. I thought I was probably beginning to hate newborn kids too![31]

The *godhbharai* is a traditional north Indian baby shower ceremony celebrated during the last trimester of pregnancy to bless the mother with a healthy baby. A common incident shared by many women struggling with infertility is that they are asked to stay away from the *godhbharai* ceremony of a close cousin or relative. This is not only insensitive, but it's also disrespectful. If you face such a situation, don't sneak or hide away and cry in the dark. Instead, stand up for yourself and deal with it in a dignified and graceful way.

For a very long time in my fertility journey, when people asked me about the 'good news', I would sneak out of the conversation with an uncomfortable smile and a looming tear. I would try to pass the evening somehow, then get back home and cry like hell. Then, one day, I mustered all my strength, looked the person who was asking me this

---

31 Interview with Sunayna Uberoy, a twenty-seven-year-old teacher.

question in the eye, and said, 'I have had three miscarriages in the past six years of marriage. We are struggling to fight infertility. And if this is the extended honeymoon, then it is of the worst kind.'

Yes, I did it. I faced my weakness and I felt strong and relieved. No more hiding, no more diplomatic answers. The person who asked the question was taken aback. She had never faced such an honest and straightforward answer. She stared at me speechlessly.

This relative *chakravyu* comes up in most Indian communities, whether you are from north or south India whether you belong to the rich or middle class. Deal with it in a way that works for you—giving them a piece of your mind, distancing yourself, having someone to shield you from them. It is important to stay away from people who bring negative energy. This journey is draining, and you are weak, both physically and emotionally. In this situation such negativity can mess with both your mind and your body.

Threat to Sexual Intimacy

Sexual intimacy is another important but unspoken stressor. One of the couples I spoke to while researching this book confessed that performing sex by the clock, with the hope of achieving conception and laden with the stress of previous failure actually killed sex for them. Infertility is perceived as a big threat to sexual identity, which leads to low self-esteem and impacts sexual functioning.

The Blame Game

During one's fertility journey, hurt, fear, and the sense of loss is so deep and intense that some couples end up blaming each other, mostly unconsciously. What begins as a discussion to figure out the next step often gets embroiled into not only blaming the partner, but also blaming the family. Heated arguments, frustration and misunderstanding keep getting added with every conversation. The result of such conversations is never conclusive. In the end, you harm your relationships and your health.

Don't play blame games. Your heart knows that your partner is not at fault. They are equally clueless and sailing in the same boat. If the blame is pointed towards someone other than your partner, then remember, it stems from a lack of sensitivity and societal indifference. It won't change easily. So be patient and don't ruin your treatment path because of what others say, do, or don't do.

The blame game is a terrible coping strategy.

Accept Your Condition and Take Action

I believe that accepting you have infertility and then taking constructive steps to tackle the situation is the best coping strategy because that will clear your path of any confusions that may arise, and you can work towards your goal. Most couples will take time to accept that they have infertility and will either stop the treatment as they lack the strength to face it or get trapped in unscientific, unproven, and even dangerous practices. By doing this, you end up harming yourself and you lose crucial time. Remember, the more you waste time, the more time you lose, and the harder it becomes to conceive as age is usually inversely proportional to conception.

Accept the situation gracefully and move on with a practical approach towards finding solutions. Be mentally strong and prepared to handle what life has thrown at you. You may adopt different strategies to accept. Some of these are:

1. **Calm acceptance**: Accepting the situation with patience and understanding. You believe that destiny has chosen a different path than what you had planned. And you undergo the process with trust.
2. **Explosive reaction**: At the onset, you simply explode, which can be in the form of anger, crying or being locked up in a room. This explosive reaction helps release the pent-up feelings of frustration. Once you cool down and begin to accept the situation, you can start planning for the new path.
3. **Resigned acceptance**: You accept your destiny but with a feeling of surrendering to the situation. Even though your heart aches, you have accepted the pain… *'Que Sera Sera/Whatever will be will be…'*

You may find acceptance in any of these three ways. How you do it is unimportant. But you should try to get done with it and move ahead. Lingering will only cause the wound to become septic. Keep yourself busy with work. However, this does not mean living in denial. Accepting infertility is a difficult situation. I've been there and I know how lonely and frustrating it can be. We have never been told or trained for a situation like this. Feeling pain is absolutely fine but going downhill isn't. You have the strength within yourself to overcome this situation.

Seek Support

Seeking support from a community that understands your situation without judgement and offers you unconditional support is a great way to cope. At Fertility Dost (www.fertilitydost.com), our peer-to-peer network of women who have either crossed over the journey of fertility or are sailing in the same boat, being mentored by professional counsellors, provides a great platform for women to make them believe that they are not alone in this journey. Most importantly, communities such as these help you realize how blessed you are when you come across how complex other women's medical journeys or family situations can be. When you meet women who are fighting endometriosis (a battle in itself), have been through three failed IVFs, are managing uncooperative husbands and in-laws, you know what to be grateful about. Comparing notes can sometimes be therapeutic.

Your situation is bad but not bad enough. So, keep your chin up and fight on!

Box 3.1: Set the Right Expectations

> 1. Know what to expect.
> 2. Understand the consequences.
> 3. Be prepared to deal with resilience.

Source: Created by the author.

Once you have coped with your initial trauma and shock, consider the above points.

4

The Different Types of Infertility
Understand Your Type

'To know what you know and what you do not know, that is true knowledge.'

— Confucius

To tackle the problem of infertility effectively, you need to have a thorough understanding of the issues, and most importantly, be mindful of what you are unable to diagnose, understand or treat. The first step in this journey of knowing is to go through multiple tests (which I discussed in Chapter 2), based on which your doctor and you will be able to conclude the type of infertility you are struggling with. This diagnosis will lead you to a particular treatment path.

However, it is not that simple! In some cases, you may be diagnosed with multiple or overlapping issues and types of infertility. These cases are the most difficult to manage.

Although it may seem like a complicated knot of problems, I am here to unravel them for you.

For now, let's look at the different types of infertility, the challenges they pose, and the solutions that are out there.

Unexplained Infertility—The Gloomiest Kind

Kasha, a thirty-one-year-old trained dancer from Chennai, says:

> Every time I visited a doctor, they would ask me to do new tests. I have done around 100–150 tests. After doing a test, I would feel really devastated. 'Why me?', I always thought. The thing is that if you have a problem, you can get the treatment for it. If there is a problem in the egg or the sperm or the uterus or whatever, you can get it sorted. But if there is no problem in anything, where do you find the solution for it? Not having the problem diagnosed is a big problem in itself. Then your family members are like, 'Kisi ne kokh bandhi hogi ya kisi ne tona kiya hoga [Someone must have done black magic]'.[32]

Unexplained fertility is the most defeating kind. When even after multiple tests, fertility experts are unable to ascertain the reason for a miscarriage, implantation failure, or the core reason for the inability of a couple to take the pregnancy to

---

32 Interview with Kasha, a thirty-one-year-old dancer, Chennai.

full term then, it is simply called 'unexplained infertility'. This kind of infertility is an emotional rollercoaster ride and takes a toll even on the strongest minds.

I had unexplained infertility. First, I was unable to come to terms with the fact that I had infertility, and then, the term 'unexplained infertility' just made things so much worse. Why couldn't my issue be explained? It was utterly bizarre. The many rounds of tests made me feel like a guinea pig. There was not a single red flag in the tests for us, and yet, I would still have a miscarriage. I endured this for three years. I would get pregnant and feel at the top of the world, confident that I had magically defeated the so-called unexplained infertility. Then, in the early term of pregnancy, I would have to painfully let go of the pregnancy after a tumultuous six to eight weeks. Along with the heartache and frustration, what followed was the even more painful second half of the year when doctors tried to figure out why the miscarriage happened. Doctors use the traditional method of using low-cost and low-intervention investigation and treatment procedures by trying stimulation; first with medicines, then with IUI, and lastly, going for IVF.

When I asked them what had gone wrong, I received a standard orchestrated response: 'All your parameters were fine. Your pregnancy should have gone through. We don't know how this happened. We will do a few more tests and make sure that next time everything goes right.'

I believed their reasoning the first time. The second time, I took it with a pinch of salt. By the third time, I was angry, frustrated, humiliated, with a self-esteem that had hit rock bottom. I knew that this problem wasn't going away. I was going around in circles, and there seemed no way to break this cycle.

The worst part of unexplained infertility is that it doesn't happen at once. It is a long-drawn-out process of tests, investigations, diagnoses and repeat. It is this medical frustration that is overwhelming. So, expectation management and constant reality checks are crucial. As a result of the lack of evidence, many couples with unexplained infertility endure (and even request) expensive, potentially hazardous, and often unnecessary treatments.[33]

PCOS Infertility—The Lingering Kind

Twenty-eight-year-old Anitha from Chennai is an Army officer's wife. She is a corporate management professional. In the initial years after marriage, Anitha wanted to hold onto her job and concentrate on work so she had decided to postpone her pregnancy. During that time, she was also detected with PCOD and started treatment for it. Six years later, she decided to have a baby but could not get pregnant. Her doctor suggested that PCOD could be a cause. However, her PCOD was not so severe that it would hamper pregnancy. Since they could not figure out the issue,

---

33 The Thessaloniki ESHRE/ASRM-Sponsored PCOS Consensus Workshop Group, 'Consensus on Infertility Treatment Related to Polycystic Ovary Syndrome', *Fertility and Sterility* 89, no. 3 (2008), pp. 505–22, available at https://sci-hub.se/10.1016/j.fertnstert.2007.09.041.

Anitha decided to opt for IVF. Her doctor told her that she was not infertile and that she could get naturally pregnant after the PCOD was resolved. However, due to parental pressure, she decided to opt for IVF.

One in every five women in India suffers from PCOS, which usually begins in adolescence.[34] It is aptly known as the 'hidden epidemic'. In brief, PCOS is an ovulatory dysfunction which impacts periods, hormones, metabolism, egg quality and reproduction. Often, initial symptoms manifest in the form of period issues, facial hair, obesity, and uncontrollable mood swings.

PCOS is usually not treated or managed well at the time it surfaces due to a lack of awareness and heavy social taboo around talking about 'periods'. This, then, leads to fertility issues at a later stage. However, the good news is that PCOS infertility is comparatively easier to manage because it is a lifestyle issue and about 70 per cent of the illness can be managed with holistic treatment.

To help break it down simply, there are three major problems associated with PCOS:

1. **Pressure on egg quality**: Every woman is born with a certain number of eggs and during every period cycle, a few of these eggs are discarded. In the case of PCOS, because periods are irregular and hormones are

---

34 Bhumika Pruthi, 'One in Five Indian Women Suffers from PCOS', *The Hindu*, 26 September 2019, available at https://www.thehindu.com/sci-tech/health/one-in-five-indian-women-suffers-from-pcos/article29513588.ece.

massively fluctuating, it puts immense pressure on the egg reserve and egg quality. So, when you finally try to conceive, this becomes a sore point.
2. **Hormonal disturbance**: Conception requires your hormones to be in perfect balance. PCOS is known for messing with your hormones and that, too, from a young age. So, in your late twenties or early thirties, when you try for pregnancy, much damage has already been caused. Now reversing this hormonal imbalance will require time and patience, but if you are at a point where you don't wish to delay pregnancy further, it becomes a complex proposition. You want to get pregnant but it will take some time to manage PCOS. The more you delay pregnancy, the egg quality diminishes further. It becomes a Catch-22 situation.

PCOS infertility takes time to resolve. You have to be patient and also be extremely vigilant. But the good news is that since in most cases a woman is aware of her PCOS and mindful that it might lead to a situation like this, the acceptance is easier and faster.

All you need to do now is get that perfect window to conceive, which can be achieved by combining medicine and alternative treatments like Ayurveda, acupuncture and naturopathy. You must sincerely and effectively work on lifestyle modification before entering the treatment phase with PCOS infertility. This will manifold improve your treatment efficacy.

Obesity + PCOS = Infertility

Obesity and PCOD are a deadly combination, often escalating into infertility. This combination is believed to impact the metabolic, hormonal and reproductive system, and there is also the chance of it escalating into Type 2 diabetes and hypertension. So as a first line of treatment, doctors usually recommend weight loss. Diet, exercise and lifestyle modifications are ideal ways to negate this equation. Weight loss before infertility treatment is known to improve ovulation rates in women with PCOS.[35, 36]

Clomiphene citrate (CC), a medicine, remains the treatment of first choice for the induction of ovulation in anovulating women with PCOS. The cost of the medication is low, the oral route of administration is patient-friendly, there are relatively few adverse effects, little ovarian response

---

[35] L.J. Moran, M. Noakes, P.M. Clifton, L. Tomlinson, C. Galletly and R.J. Norman, 'Dietary Composition in Restoring Reproductive and Metabolic Physiology in Overweight Women with Polycystic Ovary Syndrome', *The Journal of Clinical Endocrinology and Metabolism* 88, no. 2 (2003), pp. 812–19, available at https://academic.oup.com/jcem/article/88/2/812/2845309?login=false.

[36] R. Pasquali, C. Pelusi, S. Genghini, M. Cacciari and A. Gambineri, 'Obesity and Reproductive Disorders in Women', *Human Reproductive Update* 9, no. 4 (2003), pp. 359–72, available at https://academic.oup.com/humupd/article/9/4/359/737350?login=false.

monitoring is required, and abundant clinical data are available regarding the safety of the drug.[37]

Women with PCOS might not even need IVF treatment, in most cases. Lifestyle management and basic ovulation induction might just do the trick.

Diminishing Ovarian Reserve—The Shocking Kind

Most women hate having periods—that irritating, messy and painful time of the month. But despite the pain, we know that as long as our periods happen, everything is fine with our reproductive health. Then, imagine, how you'd feel when the doctor tells you that your ovarian reserve is diminishing, and you have fewer number of eggs? 'But doctor I always get my periods on time and even the flow is normal!' That's the standard response of women who are detected with a diminishing ovarian reserve as the primary cause of their fertility issues.

We are born with only a certain number of eggs. As women, we need good eggs to conceive. Our ovarian reserve is a marker of our biological clock window. AMH is the test that confirms the ovarian reserve, but it is usually done quite late in one's pre-conception journey.

I strongly believe that the assessment of ovarian reserve should be done on a regular basis from one's late twenties, even if you are unmarried. This is so that you can focus

---

[37] C. Farquhar, 'Endometriosis', *British Medical Journal* 334, no. 7587 (2007), pp. 249–53, available at https://www.jstor.org/stable/20506284.

on your career and respond to your parents' query/subtle taunts with appropriate logic and proof.

> 'Shaadi kab karogi? Jyada late karogi aur phir bacchey nahi honge to phir mujhe mat bolna [When will you get married? If you delay and then have problems while having kids then don't come running to me].'
>
> 'Mainey AMH test karwaya hai [I have done AMH test], my ovarian reserve is fine, and I still have five more years before it begins to diminish. So, chill mom! I will get married, have kids, and a happy family, too.'

While this might seem farfetched now, it is my vision for the future that every girl is aware, empowered and proactive about her health.

There are two conflicting views by experts (fertility doctors and alternative practitioners) on diminishing ovarian reserve and fertility:

1. **Nothing can be done**: Just like you can't revive someone once they are dead, this section believes that nothing can be done about a diminished ovarian reserve. So, you have to work around the issue, and an egg donor IVF cycle works like magic in such cases, given that your other parameters are mostly good. However, many couples go through a major ethical and emotional conflict when it comes to egg donor IVF cycle. More about egg donor treatment methodology in Chapter 7.

2. **You just need one egg**: This section of doctors believes that all you need to conceive is just one egg and that should not be difficult, given that you still have a reserve (even if it is on the diminishing side). It is said that through some planning and lifestyle changes, you can improve the quality of your eggs.[38] One of the effective protocols for women with diminishing ovarian reserve is a natural IVF cycle, which is basically a low dose IVF, where the focus is on the body producing eggs by natural stimulation, with minimal help of artificial stimulation (hormone injections). The logic here is that each IVF cycle leads to a rapid depletion of the ovarian reserve, which is mostly a side effect of IVF injections. However, a natural IVF cycle, which has a comparatively lower dosage of medicines, can minimize the depreciating impact on the eggs. However, on the flip side, you will have to undergo multiple rounds of the stimulation cycle for a period of three to six months.

Recurrent Miscarriages—The Frustrating Kind

Thirty-year-old Radhika from Bhopal says:

> It was real; I had a 'missed' miscarriage halfway through the first term which was discovered only in the eleventh week scan. The doctors had to clean

---

[38] Rebecca Fett, *It Starts with the Egg* (Miami, FL: Franklin Fox Publishing LLC, March 2014).

it up with a D&C procedure. I was so deluded and so attached to 'that feeling of being pregnant' that I asked the doctors to show me 'that' before giving it away in the lab for a biopsy.[39]

In this scenario, you are able to conceive easily and naturally, but the problem is in taking it to full term. It is an agonizing experience. Also, because you would be conceiving naturally, you continue to visit your gynae instead of a fertility expert. The dilemma is understandable and accentuated by a mindset that follows social norms. Your delay in meeting a fertility expert causes much harm. What looks like a benign miscarriage with the 'ho jata hai kabhi-kabhi' [sometimes it happens]' attitude, is actually indicative of deeper troubles.

When I had my first miscarriage, a relative nonchalantly said that she had seen me wearing a heeled sandal during pregnancy, which could have been a reason for my miscarriage. So, the next time I conceive, I should avoid wearing heels and I'll be able to see the pregnancy to the full term. If only things were that simple! But the truth is that, that statement got stuck in my mind and I actually stopped wearing heels for the longest time, believing this to be true, even during my non-pregnancy time, to punish myself. I had five miscarriages. I can't express in words how devastated I felt.

Genetic anomalies are usually behind recurrent miscarriages, and so it becomes even more difficult to investigate and pinpoint a reason. Also, because you are

---

39 Interview with Radhika, a thirty-year-old resident, Bhopal.

able to conceive naturally but with a risk to get or not to get pregnant becomes a medico-ethical issue. To get pregnant you might have to stop getting pregnant for a while and assess the cause. Truly ironic!

Male Infertility—The Taboo Kind

Let's now turn to the elephant in the room.

We have been conditioned to believe that if the cause of infertility lies with the woman, it is digestible, but if it lies with the man, then it's unimaginable. There are different kinds of men and varying degrees of relationship dynamics within couples, so I am not going to fall into stereotyping, but the hard truth is that in most cases, male infertility is a big setback on the perceptions, relationship dynamics and treatment.

Many women have confided in me that it was almost impossible to convince their male partner to go for a basic sperm test, which is the first step in fertility treatment. Again, when most of them were finally convinced to take the sperm test, they did it to prove their masculinity (in numbers) and put a full stop to the uncomfortable discussion. They'd earn bragging rights if the reports were good, but if the opposite were true, then accepting and moving on would become another war both inside (between the couple and inside their brains) and outside (cutting across societal taboos and built-up perceptions of masculinity).

The good news is that male infertility (except a few like azoospermia) is relatively easier to manage. Sperm quality, quantity and morphology can be managed through lifestyle modifications, antibiotic medicines (to do away with any infections) and washing sperms through IUI or intracystoplasmic sperm injection (ICSI)–IVF methodology (where sperms are washed and carefully selected to get the best lot). If you have a husband who is understanding and cooperative, you're very lucky.

Endometriosis—The Painful Kind

Shilpi Srivastava, a thirty-two-year-old woman from Jaipur, who has been married for seven years, five of which have already been consumed by fertility struggle, says:

> One day, I woke up with a mild pain in my abdomen. Even though I tried hard to avoid it, focusing on my daily schedule, it turned into a stabbing, thrashing pain. I immediately went to a doctor. I was not aware that it was going to be the start of a new painful chapter in my life. I was diagnosed with endometriosis, which damaged and blocked my fallopian tubes for life. The treatment for endometriosis took a year, then the anti-tubercular treatment (ATT), and then, I turned towards IVF. Till now I have been through one IUI, two IVF, and four frozen embryo transfers, with no result.[40]

---

40 Interview with Shilpi Srivastava, a thirty-two-year-old woman, Jaipur.

What is Endometriosis?

Endometriosis is defined as the presence of functioning uterine glands in any internal parts outside the uterus—fallopian tubes, ovaries, cervix, vagina, urinary bladder, and in rare cases, even in the lungs and liver. These implants react to hormonal changes, which leads to tissue build-up each month, which in turn break down and cause bleeding. But they have no way of leaving the body, and therefore, result in internal bleeding and inflammation.

Here are the symptoms of endometriosis:

1. Heavy periods.
2. Presence of fibroids.
3. Frequent abdominal pain.
4. Endometrium lining is affected and usually becomes bulky.
5. Fallopian tubes get damaged or blocked.
6. Pelvic anatomy gets distorted.
7. Eggs in the ovaries might also get affected due to endometriosis.

The most dangerous aspect of endometriosis is that it typically takes approximately seven-and-a-half years from the time the symptoms show up till the time the condition is actually diagnosed.[41]

---

41 Hudson N. The missed disease? Endometriosis as an example of 'undone science'. Reprod Biomed Soc Online. 2021 Aug 13;14:20-27. doi: 10.1016/j.rbms.2021.07.003. PMID: 34693042; PMCID: PMC8517707.

As per research, 'An estimated 25–50 per cent of women with infertility have endometriosis and around 30–50 per cent of women with endometriosis have infertility.'[42] For us these numbers only mean that if you, too, have endometriosis and infertility then you are not alone.

Think of endometriosis as a spider web over your uterus, affecting its normal reproductive functions. Endometriosis-led infertility is usually the most painful kind, primarily because endometriosis itself is an extremely uncomfortable condition.

The bad news is that medical science doesn't have enough knowledge about endometriosis or any permanent solution for it. In fact, there isn't any conclusive blood test that can diagnose endometriosis. If you have endometriosis, then doctors often suggest that you don't delay your pregnancy, as fibroids tend to grow and complicate the issue.

The good news is that endometrial growth is not malignant in most cases; these are normal tissues growing away from the normal location. Laparoscopic treatment helps diagnose the extent of cysts and also clears them out. This temporarily reduces period discomfort and gives couples a good window to plan pregnancy either naturally or through IVF (whichever works in your case).

---

42 M.L. Macer and H.S. Taylor, 'Endometriosis and Infertility: A review of the Pathogenesis and Treatment of Endometriosis-Associated Infertility', *Obstetrics and Gynaecology Clinics of North America* 39, no. 4 (2012), pp. 535–49.

Shveta Suri, a thirty-five-year-old woman from Gurugram, recounts:

> Until the IVF treatment, the doctors kept telling us that everything is fine in the scans, and there is nothing that they can put a finger on. The diagnosis was: there is a word for when nothing is showing, and nothing is known—unexplained. The reasons for my infertility were unexplained until then. That's what they said. But the IVF cycle had failed. I experienced many period-related problems; pain, clots, and back pain. That's when the doctors said that I may have endometriosis. We had already failed one IVF cycle when I found out that I have endometriosis. This is when I told the doctors that things aren't okay, and they may have to investigate further. It was quite a dampener.[43]

Genetic—The Confusing Kind

Infertility caused due to genetic abnormalities is difficult because it costs time, money and effort to diagnose and treat. Genetic reasons are identified mostly in two types of cases:

1. **Secondary infertility** is where you already have a child who has some genetic issues and now you are trying for a second child. So, this time you want to be

---

[43] Interview with Shveta Suri, a thirty-five-year-old woman, Gurugram.

better equipped, and therefore, genetic counselling and screening are a must.
2. **Multiple IVF failure and no conclusive reason behind it** suggests genetic reasons, which is seen as a strong reason.

Genetic issues are identified much later in the journey. Mostly, unexplained infertility and recurrent failures might hint towards genetic reasons. Interestingly, genetic issues can lie either with one of the partners or with the embryo, which means when the sperm and the egg come together to form an embryo, following which an anomaly occurs, thereby leading to implantation failure.

Secondary Infertility

If you already have one child but are facing conception issues when trying for the second child, it is called secondary infertility. According to prevalent societal myth, people find it confounding that they have infertility even when the first child was conceived and delivered normally. 'Approximately, 8 per cent of currently married women suffered from infertility in India and most of them were secondary infertile (5.8 per cent)', according to a research study.[44]

---

[44] S. Sarkar and P. Gupta, 'Socio-Demographic Correlates of Women's Infertility and Treatment Seeking Behaviour in India', *Journal of Reproduction and Infertility* 17, no. 2 (2016), pp. 123–32, available at https://ww.ncbi.nlm.nih.gov/pmc/articles/PMC4842234/.

If you wish to have a second child, then get yourself checked thoroughly. Secondary infertility is real and affects many.

It is quite possible that you might end up being diagnosed with more than one type of infertility, and that is quite common. First, don't feel overwhelmed and scared. Second, understand that infertility is a couple's problem. Use this as an opportunity to work together and be more empathic in your relationship.

Box 4.1: Takeaway Points

- Don't panic if you have more than one type of infertility.
- Use the knowledge about the right type of infertility to find the right-fit treatment path.
- Work on it together as a couple with empathy.

Source: Created by the author.

5

IUI

The First Step

YOU DON'T JUMP INTO IVF RIGHT AWAY. THERE IS A hierarchical process in the fertility treatment journey unless the diagnosis is conclusive. Some of the diagnoses are issues like fully blocked fallopian tubes, very poor egg reserve (low AMH), or advanced male fertility problems (azoospermia or similar conditions). In such cases, you should unhesitatingly go for IVF.

Since this a non-invasive procedure, IUI is generally recommended before proceeding to explore other methods of artificial insemination.

IUI is generally opted for when the sperm cannot go through the cervix for any reason. So, in cases of low sperm count or problems with sperm mobility, this procedure directly introduces the best sperm inside the uterus, thus increasing the probability of pregnancy. Also, this can be used for women who have semen allergy, unexplained infertility issues, or a cervical mucus problem.

In general, IUI can be beneficial in cases where the sperm needs a little nudge to fertilize the egg, or when the uterus needs to be made ready to accept the sperm without damaging it.

IUI is usually not successful for:

1. Women with severe endometriosis.
2. Women with pelvic adhesions.
3. Blocked fallopian tubes.
4. Previous pelvic infections.

When Can IUI Help You Conceive?

IUI works in cases when the couple has any of the following medical condition(s):

1. **Unexplained infertility issues:** In such cases, doctors have no choice but to follow the hierarchical process of treatment, which basically means starting with a low dosage and lowest intervention treatment process, assessing the effect, and then increasing the dosage one step at a time.
2. **Hostile cervical problems:** This leads to painful sex or an inability to have sex.
3. **A cervical scar:** This blocks the passage of the sperm.
4. **PCOS, after it is treated with medication:** If PCOS infertility is not responding to medicines, then

it is favourable to monitor follicular growth (done through repeated ultrasound), give ovulation-enhancing medicines, and use IUI to time the process better, as timing is the only roadblock to conception in such cases.
5. **Thick cervical mucus:** When a woman starts to ovulate, the cervical mucus becomes wet and slippery which helps the sperms to swim up easily. However, in some women, mostly due to hormal imbalance, the cervical mucus continues to be thick, which makes it difficult for the sperms to reach their right destination hurdling fertilization.
6. **Other reasons:** For instance, couples are unable to have sex during the natural ovulation cycle due to hectic work schedules or stay away from each other for long periods.
7. **Or, when your male partner has:**
   - Low sperm motility.
   - Low sperm count.
   - Ejaculation problems.
   - Impotence.
   - Varicose issue (veins that hold the testicles, enlarge hindering the sperm outflow making it impossible to conceive with no or less sperms being ejaculated).
8. **Or, in the case of same-sex couples.**

How Is IUI Procedure Performed?

The IUI procedure starts with collecting your blood samples and undergoing an ultrasound test to check your condition. If everything looks good, your IUI will be scheduled just before you start ovulating. This process is called natural IUI cycle. There is also a slight variation of this process, which is called the stimulated IUI cycle, wherein the ovulation process is stimulated using medications/injections to enhance the growth and maturity of egg follicles. Before inseminating the uterus with the sperm, you will be administered human chorionic gonadotropin (HCG) shots, generally twenty-four hours before the procedure, to increase chances of insemination.

On the day of the process, the sperm is prepared and chosen by the process of sperm washing, where a wash solution is added to the ejaculated sperms and then put into the centrifuge to produce concentrated and improved sperms for insemination. A catheter containing the sperm is then placed inside the uterus through the cervix. Generally, you are asked to lie horizontally for a few minutes after the procedure is performed.

And then, it is done! Be patient for two weeks and wait for the sperm to do its job.

After two weeks, you will be asked to take a pregnancy test at home, or you can do a check-up at the hospital, too, to see if the procedure has been fruitful.

IUI is a non-invasive treatment. You may feel a little uncomfortable when the catheter is inserted into your uterus, but it will be painless.

After the IUI procedure, the cervical mucus is loosened, and the catheter comes out easily, so you may feel wet, but that doesn't mean that the sperm has come out, and it is no reason to panic.

Doctors will ask you to lie down for a few minutes after the procedure, but post the process, there is no need to lie down or rest too much. You can go about your normal routine. However, you should be mindful and avoid extreme heavy tasks like lifting or hardcore exercises.

IUI is a safe procedure. You may experience minor cramps or bleeding after the procedure.

Ensure that the sperm is screened properly and is cleaned of any infection before being inserted into the uterus. Mostly, doctors prescribe medicines for the male partner as well to enhance effectiveness and reduce infections, if any. It is important to conduct a clean procedure, as there may be possibilities of infection if the sperm is not screened properly.

In cases of advanced male fertility issues, IUI with a sperm donor is advised.

IUI Treatment Cost

The cost of IUI is lower as compared to IVF. The typical cost of IUI procedures in India is between Rs 4,000 and Rs 15,000, depending on the place where you get it done, as well as your age and medical health. Even if you require just one cycle, you can expect to spend approximately Rs 10,000 extra as a doctor will do an ultrasound and other tests to initiate IUI treatment. So, factor in that cost as well while planning for IUI.

Table 5.1: IUI Costs in Different Metropolitan Cities in India

Location	IUI Cost*
Delhi	Rs 6000 to Rs 10,000
Mumbai	Rs 8,000 to Rs 15,000
Bengaluru	Starts From Rs 8,000
Hyderabad	Starts from Rs 7,000
Kolkata	Starts from Rs 6,000

Note: *These prices are indicative only.
Source: Created by the author.

IUI Success Rate in India

For a woman below the age of thirty-five, chances of pregnancy through IUI are 10–20 per cent, while for a woman between the age group of thirty-five to forty, the chances are 10 per cent. For women above the age of forty, the chances reduce to 5 per cent. The success rate of IUI is lower than the success rate of IVF.

Table 5.2: IUI Success Rate in Women Based on Age Group

Age of Woman	Successful Implantation/ Pregnancy Rate* (in Per Cent)	Healthy Baby Delivery Rate (in Per Cent)
Between twenty and thirty years	20	15

Age of Woman	Successful Implantation/ Pregnancy Rate* (in Per Cent)	Healthy Baby Delivery Rate (in Per Cent)
Between thirty and thirty-five years	15	11
Between thirty-five and thirty-nine years	14	10
Forty plus years	5	3

Note: *Indicative numbers collected and collated after interviewing multiple IUI doctors/clinics in India.
Source: Created by the author.

Box 5.1: Things You Need to Keep in Mind

- Avoid having sex/ejaculation two to three days before IUI is done to ensure best quality sperms.
- You can have sex after the IUI process to increase chances of implantation.
- You don't need to take bedrest after the IUI process. Just avoid a heavy or hectic schedule.
- Do the pregnancy test after two weeks.
- Take home cooked healthy diet.

Source: Created by the author.

Home IUI Kits

These days you can even do IUI at home. There are many IUI kits available in the market along with apps to guide you through the process. However, you may require a nurse to facilitate the process. Such kits are a boon for couples with hectic work schedules. However, these kits can only help you with natural IUI cycles. As they are quite recent, I can't comment on the success rate of home IUI kits.

Advanced Tests When IUI Fails

If your IUI fails, then most doctors will move to the next stage of advanced tests. These tests are expensive, time-consuming, and painful in some cases. However, these tests are critical to understand why the IUI process isn't working and mostly to build up a cogent case to move you up in the ladder of fertility treatments aka the IVF stage.

Diagnostic tests are an important part of the fertility journey. When the journey gets tough, so do the tests. Advanced fertility tests like HSG, diagnostic laparoscopy, or biopsy for tuberculosis are invasive and often require day admission.

They are necessary evils in this process and can be frustrating at all levels. You hope that the test is conclusive so that you know exactly what you need to do to lead you towards your desired path of motherhood, but many questions and ifs and buts can arise.

More often than not, these tests are inconclusive and lead to another set of tests, and endless waiting with a vague idea of a treatment plan to follow. Well, there are certain things you can't change or control, except walking the path with dignity, patience and grit.

However, there are a few things you can do to ensure that you navigate this stage properly. Some unethical clinics or doctors might ask you to undergo a test that might not be really necessary, is expensive, and does not directly impact your specific line of treatment. Remember, such people take advantage of your desperation. You must steer clear of such practices. Ensure that the tests are conducted properly, and you are fully informed and prepared for them.

I was in Chennai and got a consultation appointment with a very senior fertility specialist almost after a month. Already overwhelmed when I entered her chamber, within two minutes, she suggested that I go for the HSG test and that it would have to be done right away. This is a test which includes inserting a chemical dye through your vagina. Not only was it expensive, but I wasn't prepared either as I had come in for just consultation. I requested if I may undergo it the next day, but they gave some weird reason, and I had to undergo the test at 9 p.m. in the night right after the consultation. It was a horrific experience.

As most fertility tests are hormone-related and period cycle-dependant, it is extremely essential that protocol and timings are followed to a tee; otherwise, you will end up retesting or being misdiagnosed.

Also, don't hesitate to ask questions and don't be intimidated by your doctor.

Ask Questions, Ask Questions, Ask Questions— That's the Mantra!

If your doctor is not answering properly or satisfactorily, then it is time to rethink your doc. Also, know when to stop the IUI process.

As IUI is cheap and non-invasive, unlike IVF, couples tend to continue with multiple and mostly unnecessary rounds of IUI. Having hope is good but know where to draw the line. If IUI is not working for you after three cycles, then it is time to scrutinize it closely. Remember, you are wasting precious time here as age inversely impacts conception.

Box 5.2: Key Points to Remember

- Follow the timings properly. Do your tests during the right time in your ovulation/period cycle.
- Ask your doctor questions. For example, why do I need this test? What will it achieve?
- Read about and understand the tests.
- Not knowing what to expect causes stress and stress impacts the treatment.
- Know when to stop IUI.

Source: Created by the author.

6

IVF
The Basics

'They did an ultrasound and explained that I needed to self-inject for a number of weeks, stimulating the eggs. Then I'd return and they'd be harvested. "We hope for a good crop", said the doctor. The language made it sound so simple, like plucking watermelons from a patch. I went in for my second egg harvesting session. I learned how to self-inject and was handed a bunch of requisitions for blood work. I looked at the forms—oh, all these forms—and felt immediately exhausted. In the past few months, there had been too many choices, too many decisions and about my body and my future. I just wanted to be cosy and slovenly at home, to scrunch deeper into my blanket and dream. I was tired of injections, of being poked and prodded.' – Lisa Ray, *Close to the Bone*[45]

---

45 Lisa Ray, *Close to the Bone* (Gurugram, Haryana: HarperCollins India, , 2019).

Actress and model Lisa Ray so humanely brings out her fight with her cancer treatment! At this particular point in her life, while she was in the thick of her treatment, Lisa decided to freeze her eggs. Her frustration resonates with anyone going through life-altering treatments. She rightly points out that even if you are surrounded by all these people offering support and kindness, cancer (in our context, fertility) is a 'very singular, very individual, very lonely journey', and also a very long journey.[46]

You will be shrouded by a fog of conflict for most part of the journey—conflict both inside and outside, conflict with people and your surroundings, conflict about the right treatment path. There will be so many decisions that the process is bound to change you forever. In hindsight, I can say with confidence that the fertility journey changes you for good, teaches life lessons like humility, gratitude, empathy, to love your imperfections with dignity, and most importantly, to trust yourself.

Begin the Journey with a Sense of Trust

On paper, the process of IVF is simple. Eggs and sperms are fertilized in a lab to make an embryo, which is then transferred into the woman's uterus vaginally for implantation. The scientific understanding of the process is not difficult to comprehend; rather, it is the emotional

---

46 Lisa Ray, *Close to the Bone* (Gurugram, Haryana: HarperCollins India, 2019).

burden of IVF which confounds, stresses and is painful to manage.

The biggest reason for IVF failure is *scare*, which is borne out of not knowing what to expect and *hoping for a miracle*, thereby setting the wrong expectation. You must remember this—there are no miracles in this journey. *In fact, anything that is posed as a miracle in IVF is simply a marketing gimmick.*

You don't get sent for the IVF process right away; there are many procedures, decisions and trials before that decision. This chapter aims to give you an overview of the whole process in a hierarchical step-by-step manner. You might get pregnant at any stage and move out of the journey with a baby in your arms, or sadly, you may continue till the fag end (discussed in detail in Chapters 7 and 12). Decision-making is a critical component of the fertility journey, and you can make good decisions only if you are thorough with the basics.

Breaking Myths Around IVF

Often women undergoing infertility treatments reach a stage where they have to take a leap of faith—a jump towards IVF. This is an extremely critical phase of the infertility journey, usually unnerving and emotionally draining. Preparing one's mind for IVF is no easy task. Couples hide their fear under excuses like, 'We are so young; we don't need IVF' or 'We will just wait it out.'

The reason behind this fear is the lack of correct knowledge about IVF. Add to it the mythical IVF stories that a relative will tell you (apparently whose brother's-wife's-mami's daughter-in-law had gone for IVF). This section dispels myths about IVF and gives you precise information to help you prepare for IVF by thinking right and making an informed decision.

Recurrent Miscarriages Mean You Don't Need IVF

Unexplained miscarriage in the first trimester can happen once or be a recurrent phenomenon. When three or more pregnancies are lost, it is called recurrent miscarriages.[47]

Recurrent miscarriages are a frustrating problem for the affected couple.

The thing about miscarriages is that it keeps the hopes alive. Medically, the truth is that you can conceive absolutely normally and take it to full term even after one miscarriage. This is also a predominant social thought.

In my case, I had three miscarriages one after the other. The year would start with hope and doctor visits. I would conceive naturally, take the pregnancy to around seven to nine weeks when 'no heartbeat' would be declared, followed by a D&C. The second half of the year would go in fighting depression and investigating the reason behind the miscarriage. Ultimately, two theories would surface:

---

[47] H.B. Ford and D.J. Schust, 'Recurrent Pregnancy Loss: Etiology, Diagnosis, and Therapy', *Obstetrics and Gynecology* 2, no. 2 (2009), pp. 76–83, available at https://www.ncbi.nlm.nih.gov/pmc/articles/PMC2709325/.

1. **Medical:** No conclusive reason for the miscarriage.
2. **Social:** As long as you are conceiving naturally, there is no problem. It happens, and you should try again. Sometimes it would be the fault of my hectic job, while at other times, it would be my high heels or that I wasn't eating properly.

My miscarriages kept happening and I stayed stuck in this loop even when one of the doctors told me that I needed to up the treatment game and that I might have infertility. I rejected this thought because I felt that I was conceiving naturally and was endorsed by my comfort circle of family. I thought that artificial insemination or the IVF path was not for me and it was just a matter of time before I conceived and took it to full term.

IVF is for Older Women

The reason why there are more older women going for IVF treatment is that they wait and wait till they have exhausted all the other options. As it is, infertility diagnosis and treatment are time-consuming, and then, couples deter going for IVF till they have absolutely no options left, thus diminishing their success chances even further. Remember, success through IVF depends on a complex combination of various factors, and not just on your age.

If you are also hesitant to take the jump towards IVF only because you think you are young and IVF is for older women, then, my dear, you are losing out on precious time. If your problem behind non-conceiving or failed conceptions has been diagnosed and you have been advised to go for IVF, then don't waste time. The truth is, the younger you are, the better are your chances of a successful IVF. You would be lucky to have reached diagnosis and solution early. So, why hang about? Resolve the problem and get on with life.

Young Age = Better Egg Quality = Good Success Chances

I Will Conceive Naturally!

A lot of women tell themselves this when they are fed up with infertility, and when they are really depressed. Trust me, this is no solution. You must continue to fight. Hoping that you will conceive naturally while knowing that you have problems that require assisted technologies is naive behaviour. In life, there are no simple solutions. Also, a lot of miraculous stories you keep hearing, of natural conception after years of struggle, may not be entirely true. Many couples in India undergo IVF, surrogacy, sperm donation, egg donation or such measures in a complete hush-hush manner and then present it as natural conception (owing to societal pressures and the stigma attached to infertility treatments). So, be realistic. Acknowledge your problem, and only then you will be able to look for the right solution.

With IVF, I Will Succeed, Pakka

Wrong. IVF is no miracle treatment. It does work to solve a lot of infertility problems, but not all of them. Again, use your logic. Ask questions and set realistic expectations when one round of IVF fails. Adjust your treatment plan accordingly and try again. However, being too hopeful will lead to extreme depression if it doesn't work out. Remember, every patient is unique. It is not necessary that since your friend's IVF cycle succeeded, yours will too. Taking a balanced approach is the best. Always chalk out a Plan B to avoid messy emotional situations. There are options beyond IVF like adoption or surrogacy that might work for you. Be mentally prepared. I always say, 'Hope for the best but be prepared for the worst.'

Don't jump into IVF the moment your doctor utters the word. Set your expectations right. It is no miracle treatment. You need to prepare your body and mind to get the best out of this treatment. Take time and make efforts to prepare yourself properly. If IVF needs to be done, it needs to be done. Prepare thoroughly for IVF while keeping your mind open. Take good decisions. Soon, you will find joy in life through your little one, and then it won't matter what route you took.

Let us now focus on preparing well for IVF.

When Do You Need IVF?

This is a complicated question. I'm going to help you decode it with some pointers. Just remember, IVF can vary from situation to situation, so it totally depends on your context. Use this discussion in the context of your medical history and journey.

First, and most importantly, *trust your gut feeling*. You will know. Your mind will fight the idea, but your heart will know when it's time for IVF.

As per general protocol that is followed, after three to six rounds of IUI, doctors move to the next level of treatment, which is IVF.

However, in some cases, when there is a clear diagnosis (like a full tubal blockage), then it makes sense to start IVF without wasting any more time.

Still, I would say that three IUIs are more than enough. There is no point stretching beyond that. I have seen cases where couples were made to go for eight to ten IUIs. It is a complete waste of time, money and hope for them. This usually happens in smaller towns where clinics prefer to keep the patient for as long as possible. These are simple and naïve couples who stay put with all their hopes pinned on the clinics. Limited awareness, high desperation of the couples, the monopolistic attitude of fertility clinics and social stigma, all bundled together, have an adverse effect on the treatment path, leading to a long-drawn, and mostly unrequired struggle with infertility.

The Golden Rule with IVF is Preparedness

Ask yourself if you are prepared to undergo IVF; not just financially, but also emotionally and physically. Never jump into it just because your doctor said so or you have a family wedding to which you'd like to bring your child to avoid more taunts and questions. I'm not joking here! Trust me, I hear so many reasons of going for IVF immediately, except the right ones.

Check if You are Emotionally Fit for IVF

Did you know that when IVF had just started in 1978, a woman had to go through an emotional preparedness test, and if she failed that, she wasn't allowed to go for IVF? However, today, clinics tend to overlook this aspect when it comes to the business of IVF. Nor are the patients aware of this critical aspect. They naively believe—pay the money, trust the doctor and next thing you know is a successful IVF.

Stress, anxiety and depression will have a subtle but adverse impact on the IVF process.

It is natural for you to feel stress and anxiety because the IVF process is, in itself, intimidating. The trick is to learn how to manage stress beforehand and have a friend or professional who can help you through this phase.

Know Everything about the IVF Process

Knowing all about the process will help you be calm and prepare well. Read, ask your doctor, and prepare your mind. Also, reach out and connect with other women who have been through IVF. They will give you practical tips on the actual journey.

Preparing Your Body

I always say this to couples who reach out to me:

> 'Think about IVF like it's an IIT or IIM entrance exam. At first, you pay Rs 1,000 for the form and fill it in, but does that ensure your seat? No, right? You have to study and slog for hours before the final exam. The more you are prepared, the better are your chances of success in the entrance exam. The same rule applies for IVF.'

Just because you paid for IVF, that doesn't mean it will be successful. You will have to work towards success. To reiterate my words earlier in this chapter, there are no shortcuts or magic.

A balance of a healthy body and happy mind is optimal for successful embryo implantation and a full-term pregnancy, leading to the birth of a healthy child. Most IVF pregnancies are high-risk, and thus, have a higher risk of miscarriage or pre-term delivery.

The success rate of IVF in India is approximately 35 per cent. Thus, I can't stress enough on preparing your mind and body well not just to conceive, but also so that you are strong enough to carry the pregnancy to nine months. The ultimate aim is to have a healthy baby.

You must work on improving the endometrium lining so that implantation happens because this is another black hole where doctors can't do much and miracles of science won't work. Doctors will try their best to sort the best egg, best sperm, make the best embryo, transfer the embryo as close to the uterus as possible, work on the environment by injecting hormones, *but* whether the embryo implants or not will depend on your body's acceptability and also a bit on your luck.

You can't control luck, but you can definitely prepare your body, immunity and internal strength. We will discuss the how-tos for this in Chapter 8 For now, just remember to be mindful that you need time and a proper environment to prepare your body. Account for this while planning your IVF timeline.

Work on Your Relationships

Recognize and keep your positive relationships close to you. Try to remove any negative associations from your daily life. If you can't remove them altogether, ignore them as much as you can. Don't let their negativity impact you. Build a white wall of light around you and let nothing enter this wall.

Build your strength. You are a going to be a mother; you are more powerful than you realize. Bring that fire out.

How to Choose the Right Doctor

Rashi, a forty-year-old science teacher from Jammu, says:

> Initially all doctors are good but after two to three visits they show their true colours. There is no clear answer to anything. Every doctor tells

you different things. Few say that for fibroids one should get laparoscopy or hysteroscopy. I consulted a renowned doctor in Delhi who said that surgery might not be an option as the fibroids are too small currently. And some say it is not suggested. We are hence in a condition of confusion and we have not finalised on a doctor.[48]

Jaisnavi, a twenty-six-year-old freelancer from Kanpur, says:

I wanted to ask the doctor what she had found and if everything was okay. She only said that everything was normal and that she hadn't found anything. She should've told me if something was wrong. She never revealed any other information to me. Also, by reading the reports you cannot understand much since it's in medical jargon. She should've explained all of it to me. I even question the doctor now sometimes in my head—why did she do this and why did she do that? I used to keep googling to find information.[49]

Mandeep, a thirty-four-year-old woman from Delhi who has been trying to conceive for ten years now, says:

The doctor didn't tell me the reason for me not getting pregnant. I don't think they care. They treat us like they are treating another fever. There is a lack

---

48 Interview with Rashi, a forty-year-old teacher, Jammu.

49 Interview with Jaisnavi, a twenty-six-year-old freelancer, Kanpur.

of sensitivity. They are not invested enough. They are more involved before you sign up [for the treatment].[50]

IVF success and your comfort during this process will largely depend on the doctor or the clinic. It is of absolute importance that you decide on one that you are confident about or one that you trust.

Younger Versus Older Doctor

I believe when it comes to choosing a gynaecologist, someone who is older is better; but for IVF, the opposite is true. My logic is simple: IVF is a comparatively new field and an advanced offshoot of the department of gynaecology. The first IVF was done only in 1978.

Box 6.1: The First IVF Baby

> The world's first IVF baby, Louise Brown, was born on 25 July 1978 in the UK through the efforts of Dr Robert G. Edwards and Dr Patrick Steptoe. The world's second, and India's first IVF baby, Kanupriya, alias Durga, was born 67 days later on 3 October 1978, through the efforts of Dr Subhas Mukherjee and his two colleagues in Kolkata.

Source: Created by the author.

---

50 Interview with Mandeep, a thirty-four-year-old woman, Delhi.

The field of IVF is very dynamic. There is new research, a new procedure, and a new thesis being produced almost every day. So, you need a doctor who is abreast with the latest studies and technology and is not afraid of taking an unconventional approach.

Find Someone Who Looks at Your Case Individually

You need a doctor who studies your case individually and not like one in the herd.

I once visited a very famous IVF doctor from Bengaluru. She is so famous that people revere her like a Goddess. At her clinic, I met junior doctors, waited for hours, underwent impromptu ultrasound test and multiple blood tests for the senior doctor who won't even call you unless you get all the basic stuff done. I followed the process as dictated. Finally, after two days, we were called to the main doctor's chamber, where she truly sat like a Goddess, surrounded by her junior doctors. I took a seat, and then, the junior doctors mumbled some coded jargon into the doctor's ears, post which she said, 'Put her on that schedule.' Then, she looked at me and said, 'Everything will be fine. I have seen your case and now the junior doctors will tell you what to do.'

That was it.

I was prompted to get up and the next patient was called in. I tried to say something but was hushed and directed to walk out. Outside, I was handed a photocopied sheet of medicine and treatment routine. When I looked around, almost everyone in that room was holding the same sheet of paper. I had never felt more dejected in my life. I ran towards my car and cried to my heart's content. I was not ready to follow a herd treatment. Kid or no kid, I couldn't do this to myself. I tore the paper and never again went back to that doctor.

Someone Who is Accessible

I know doctors are busy, but compassion and warmth are must characteristics. In this world of technology, there are myriad ways in which doctors can set up a system of being accessible and approachable without disturbing their schedules.

With some doctors, we have seen that they are extremely approachable initially, but the moment the couple signs up for IVF and pays the money, they go MIA. Stay away from such doctors who 'ghost' you.

IVF is not medically a life-threatening emergency. If anything, it is a lifestyle-driven treatment and an extremely emotional one. As per an Indian Council of Medical Research (ICMR), New Delhi directive, having a counsellor at every IVF clinic is mandatory.[51]

Dr Munjaal Kapadia, Consultant Obstetrician, Gynaecologist and Infertility Specialist, from Mumbai, says:

---

51 National Guidelines for Accreditation, Supervision & Regulation of ART Clinics in India by Ministry of Health & Family Welfare, Government of India, 2005, available at https://main.icmr.nic.in/sites/default/files/art/ART_Pdf.pdf.

> If you are open and accessible, then the patients don't feel that they are cheated. You have to give them time, talk to them, take them through the process and not designate these tasks to your junior doctor. The patient comes because of your name and belief in you. And, you have to respect that sentiment of the patients.[52]

A good tip to find out if your doctor is truly accessible or not is to ask them questions, even the uncomfortable ones, and see how they respond. Do they revert with patience? Or do they snub you?

Famous Versus Not-So-Famous

Fatima, a twenty-nine-year-old art enthusiast from Lucknow, says:

> My journey has been very difficult emotionally and it has taken a toll on my health. I strongly believe mine was a case of medical negligence. The septum phase had led to multiple tests which again led to endometrium growth. And while I was seeking to improve my condition, it went from worse to worst. I realised that I would have been in a better condition had I not reached out to high profile doctors. The

---

52 Interview with Dr Munjaal Kapadia, Consultant Obstetrician, Gynaecologist and Infertility Specialist, Mumbai.

medical assistants/management team was not very helpful. They were rude with the patients and the doctor was inaccessible. The process of reaching the main doctor was very bureaucratic and inconvenient.[53]

Now, there are two types of doctors—those who are famous and those who are good. Personally, I would go with a doctor who is good but not very famous. The problem with very famous doctors is obvious:

1. **Busy**: They are extremely busy, so most of the time, you end up with a junior doctor. Even if they tell you that the procedure will be done by the famous doctor, that's rarely the case. Also, the entire IVF process rests on trust. During my frequent visits, if I don't get to interact enough with my doctor, it impacts my confidence in the operation theatre. I would like to have a familiar face around at the peak of my anxiety.
2. **Long waiting period**: Their clinics have the longest waiting period. Once, I went to a very famous doctor in Chennai. She was so famous that she had two clinics at extreme corners of the city, and she would sit in one place in the mornings and at the other in the evenings. I chose the evening slot as it was closer to my house. My appointment time, given over phone, was 9 p.m. I finally only met her at 1:30 a.m. Her waiting room was filled with half-asleep people. When I went in for the

---

53 Interview with Fatima, a twenty-nine-year-old art enthusiast, Lucknow.

consultation, I don't remember what she said; I forgot what I had to ask. All I remember was the smell of her fresh gajra, gayatri mantra playing in the background, and her crisp and pleated off-white saree, and my first thought was, 'She's so hard working!'

3. **It's a numbers game for them**: They work on numbers. So, if they see 100 cases in a month and twenty-five of them are successful, they are done for that month. Theoretically speaking. Not that they don't want your case to be successful, but they are not vested in you. It is like going to your neighbourhood grocery shop where the shopkeeper will greet you, ask you about your family, get the stuff dropped to your car, and will be generally amicable because you are an important customer for them. In a supermarket, you'll get more stuff and have more choices minus the warmth.

4. **Scare**: Most of us aren't very comfortable talking to doctors about our issues. Then imagine talking to a really famous doctor! Many women I've interacted with find famous doctors intimidating. Ultimately, you feel awed by the larger-than-life image of the doctor and don't end up speaking your mind to avoid irritating them for they seem to you to be the last beacon of hope. Yup! I have done it myself. All I could muster to ask was, 'Doctor, will I be able to conceive?' Such a useless question to ask when meeting an IVF doctor.

5. **High Hopes**: For me, this is the biggest roadblock. With a famous doctor, our hopes of a miracle increases manifold. Wrong expectations are set, which leads to painful heartbreaks, especially when the IVF fails

because only 30 per cent of IVF cycles, on an average are a success, which means 70 per cent (majority) IVF cycles are failing.[54]

Sure, famous doctors are famous because they have more experience and they have consistently given results, and most importantly, they have a workable system set up. I don't have anything against famous doctors, but I do feel that I am better off with the not-so-famous but technically good and approachable doctor because I know that this doctor will try her best to make my case successful, as every case matters to them. The doctor should have the zeal and hunger to be famous, and to do so, they need your case to be successful so that you add another feather in their progressive graph.

This is, however, an inconclusive debate, and what you choose will depend on who you are and what you want.

Decoding Success Rate as Poised by Clinics

'The success rate of any ART procedure is below 30 per cent under the best of circumstances.'

– ICMR Guidelines

---

54 N. Malhotra, D. Shah, R. Pai, H.D. Pai and M. Bankar, 'Assisted Reproductive Technology in India: A 3-Year Retrospective Analysis', *Journal of Human Reproductive Sciences* 6, no. 4 (2013), pp. 235–40, available at https://www.jhrsonline.org/article.asp?issn=0974-1208;year=2013;volume=6;issue=4;spage=235;epage=240;aulast=Malhotra.

Success rate is a critical component in choosing the IVF doctor and the clinic. The funny thing is that there is no foolproof way of getting the success rate of an IVF doctor and clinic. No clinic will claim that their success rate is less than 70 per cent, and there are no papers to prove it. No mechanism to know. When the general IVF success rate at the national level is between 30 and 35 per cent, I am completely baffled at these claims that are blatantly made. Usually, IVF centres manipulate the numbers internally and present a higher success claim than it is in reality. This happens because the government has not made it mandatory for the IVF clinics to submit their details to the government. However, things are changing for good with the introduction of the new ART Bill of 2022.

It is more of a marketing tool rather than true numbers. If every clinic has an above 70 per cent success rate, then who are these women who are crying and are stuck in infertility treatment for so many years?

Success rate is an elusive number. A better way is to look for reviews and recommendations from a trusted community. Ask people, look for an IVF support group. At Fertility Dost, this is the most frequently asked question. In fact, I started Fertility Dost to help people find the answer to this one question: 'Is this doctor/clinic good?' The intention was also to save them from the unethical gold-digging clinics.

Standalone Clinic Versus Branded Chain of IVF

Branded IVF centres with multiple clinics that have a corporate-like setup are good because they have a proper system, all accreditations are in place, an in-house embryologist is available, and the doctors or staff aren't dictators. If there is any issue or complaint, then you can raise it to the higher administration.

Standalone clinics mostly function under the name of a particular doctor who runs the show. If you choose a standalone clinic, it is mostly for the doctor. The problem with standalone clinics is that they might not have a lab or an embryologist in the clinic, but rather, they have a tie-up for these facilities. An in-house embryologist and all accreditations in place are the two non-negotiable requirements while choosing a clinic.

Embryologist — The Most Important Requirement

An embryologist is the most important person in the IVF process. They are the folks who make your babies in the lab. It is a complex process where timing, lab equipment quality, cleanliness, and a whole lot of factors matter. It is important that:

1. A clinic has an in-house embryology lab and not a tie-up with some other lab. This will jeopardize the process due to multiple handling.

2. Ensure that the embryologist is not a part-timer. To cut costs, some clinics hire visiting senior embryologists. While the juniors conduct the routine process, the senior embryologist will come in for the main task. This is done to cut down on clinic costs. However, commitment and quality become a problem in this arrangement. Timing is crucial, and you can't expect personalized attention from a visiting embryologist. Such clinics usually plan most of their egg retrieval processes (of a given month) on the same day (called batch IVF), making it easy for the embryologist to work. This arrangement, though cost-effective for the couple, runs the risk of embryo wastage. If you are already struggling with fewer number of eggs (low AMH) and are expecting to have just one to two embryos formed, you might want to speak with your embryologist.

Beware of the Unethical Market

High desperation of couples to have a baby, social taboos, and high cost of treatment have led to the mushrooming of IVF clinics that run on unethical practices.

These clinics don't have all accreditations in place, operate on blurred lines legally, make false claims, and work on your desperation.

Mixing up of sperm and eggs to increase their success rates is the most common allegation against such mushrooming clinics. Apart from this, money-trapping the couple and medical complications during the process are some of the other issues.

One of my Fertility Dost team members, Sajjitha (name changed), mother of a seven-year-old son born out of self-egg IVF cycle, recently came to know that the child is not theirs genetically. He has been diagnosed with a rare genetic medical condition; in due course of routine investigations, doctors found that the parents are not a match, and that's when they got the DNA test done. She confided in me with tears rolling down and palms pressing the forehead in desperation:

> All hell broke loose! I mean, he is my son, and he is sick. Now after seven years, one fine day I am told that he is not my son. I can't give him my tissue to save his life as I am not his mum. I can't find the egg donor as mine was a self-egg IVF cycle. I was not even told that there had been a mix-up. The clinic is not cooperating, and I can't sue as I don't want my extended family to know all this and add to our piling woes. What am I supposed to think?[55]

This incident shook me to the core. The issue in the above case is not whether the child is theirs or not; the bigger issue now is that the child's medical condition has no solution, and his condition is worsening every day. He is dying.

---

55 Interview with Sajjitha, mother of a seven-year-old son through IVF.

Therefore, you must research the clinic thoroughly before signing up for treatment. You don't want to get out of one problem and land straight into another.

Box 6.2: An Interesting Fact on IVF Clinics in India

> Did you know that there are 20,000 IVF clinics across India but merely 1500 have applied for registration with ICMR and only 390 clinics have actually completed the enrolment process?

Note: All of this will change in the new ART Bill.
Source: Created by the author.

Clinics debate that being registered with ICMR increases unnecessary paperwork without any actual benefit. The other side of the story is that clinics are hesitant of being supervised by the government regulations. Absence of stringent government regulatory measures leads to pathetic service outcome for patients. Unless the government makes registration mandatory, it will be difficult to control the quality of service at IVF clinics and price benchmarking, causing continued exploitation of couples undergoing IVF.

Choose the right clinic based on knowledge till the government draws up concrete quality control policies. There are no shortcuts in life, and in fertility treatments, there is absolutely none. Only patience and perseverance can see you through this dark tunnel to the other side.

An Overview of the IVF process

Let's begin with understanding how the basic IVF process is conducted:

Step 1 — Stimulation Phase

Ovaries are stimulated by injecting fertility medications to produce multiple eggs. This process begins with a new cycle (usually from the second day of your period) and ovulation growth is monitored closely. You are asked to come to the clinic on alternate days and in some cases almost every day.

Step 2 — Egg Retrieval

The day when eggs seem ready to mature you are injected with Human Chronic Gonadotropin (HCG) to cause the final maturation stage. This injection stimulates egg release. Egg retrieval process is conducted under general anaesthesia. It is a fifteen to thirty minutes process. Eggs are then retrieved through ultrasound whereby a hollow needle is injected into each follicle. The liquid surrounding each egg is sucked out. At the same time, your male partner is asked to provide sperm.

Step 3 — Fertilization

Post egg retrieval you are asked to go back home and rest for two to three days. Meanwhile, the lab work begins. The eggs are then fertilized in the lab, by adding sperms to it. Embryos are made.

Step 4—Embryo Transfer

It is a simple process of five to seven minutes. The embryos are placed back in the uterus after being cultured in the lab. They are placed in the uterine cavity by trans-cervical transfer where a catheter is used to negotiate through the cervix to carefully place the embryo into the uterus. This is the most crucial stage of the process. If not placed in the right location or if uterine contraction causes the embryo to shift from its location, IVF can fail.

I will talk about each of these steps in detail in Chapter 7.

The different types of IVF are nothing but a variation of this basic process.

What type of IVF is chosen for you or will work for you depends on a mix of factors—where you are in your fertility journey, medical background, age and budget.

ICSI-IVF

In normal IVF, an environment is created in the lab so that the sperm self-selects and enters the egg. This works in cases where sperm quality, especially its motility, is not that bad. In intracytoplasmic sperm injection (IVF-ICSI), a single sperm is selected and injected in the oocyte, thereby confirming fertilization. ICSI-IVF is preferred when sperm quality is on the lower side. It increases the chances of fertilization.

Mild Versus Aggressive IVF

The main difference between these two types of IVF is in the stimulation phase. Usually, the first IVF is mild, and the aim is to let your own ovulation cycle produce eggs naturally, keeping the stimulants to a minimum. This is also known as natural or low dose IVF. Cost is also on the lower side and so are the medicines. Usually, the first IVF is done following mild methodology, and if it doesn't work, the next level is aggressive IVF where the dosage of stimulation causing injections are increased. The aim is to get as many egg follicles as possible to increase probability. Needless to say, the cost of IVF in this process increases considerably.

However, a side effect of aggressive IVF is hyper-stimulation. Some women might not respond well to the stimulants. This complication is called Ovarian Hyper-Stimulation Syndrome (OHSS). Be mindful that paying extra money might not always lead towards the result.

Mild or aggressive mode of the IVF will depend on:

1. Your body's response to stimulants.
2. Number of eggs you are making normally—aggressive makes sense if you are making very few eggs.
3. Where you are in the fertility journey.

Self and Donor IVF Cycle

Self IVF cycle is one with your own egg and your own partner's sperm. Donor IVF cycle is when the egg, sperm or the embryo is someone else's—an anonymous entity. Doctors try to match the physical characteristics to some extent, and they meticulously screen for the health parameters of the donor. The donor process is completely anonymous. The recipient couple will never be told the donor's identity, and vice versa.

Donor IVF cycles can be of three types:

Egg Donor IVF

As women age, the quality and quantity of the eggs they produce decreases. Therefore, if a woman in her forties uses donor eggs, her chances of having a baby through IVF increases by about 49.6 per cent. Other scenarios are absence of ovaries, low AMH, repeated miscarriages, and chromosomal abnormality, which might require egg donor IVF cycles. In cases where at an early age a woman had to undergo chemotherapy as part of cancer treatment, she might also need this IVF protocol for procreation.

It is not a simple process. It involves intense screening and matching. There are egg banks and agencies that collect eggs, but many clinics now prefer to use fresh, unfrozen eggs. In this, the reproductive cycles of both the donor and recipient are synced, and the eggs produced are used right away.

In cases when AMH level is poor, which basically means you are not producing enough eggs or are not producing good quality eggs due to some unexplained genetic reason, egg donor IVF cycle is suggested. In this, a donor is stimulated, and their egg is retrieved. It is then fertilized with your partner's sperm and embryo is transferred into your uterus. The process is as follows:

1. Egg donors are carefully selected after intense screening and interviews.
2. Couples choosing to opt for donor eggs can select a candidate from the pool of egg donors. If the donor is available during the recipient's time frame, they are accepted.
3. The donor and the recipient's cycles are synced. While the donor is prepared for egg formation, the recipient prepares her endometrial lining for implantation (it should be at least 7 mm).
4. When the donor's eggs are developed, her eggs are retrieved using a small procedure.
5. The retrieved eggs are fertilized with the partner's sperm, and the embryos that result from it are transferred into the recipient's uterus (usually on day three or five).
6. Donors are checked to confirm that they are recovering well. The recipient is checked for pregnancy on the fourteenth day after embryo transfer via beta HCG test (a blood test).

Sperm Donor IVF

In this process, there can be two scenarios. If all the parameters of the woman are correct and sperm reports are extremely bad or there is an identified issue of azoospermia (not producing sperm), pregnancy can be achieved through IUI using donor sperm.

However, if there are some physiological issues with the female partner along with sperm issues in the male partner, sperm donor IVF process is followed.

Embryo Donor IVF

If you have:

1. Unexplained infertility.
2. More than three failed IVFs.
3. Complicated medical issues with both partners, like low ovarian reserve for the female and severe male factors like nil sperm or genetic condition.
4. Genetic anomaly in the embryo formed by self or risk of couple passing on the genetic risk to the baby.

These are some of the general situations in which you will be suggested embryo donor IVF. In this case, only the final stage of the embryo transfer will be conducted on you. Egg and sperm donors remain anonymous.

The Ethical Debate about Donor IVF

Sumita, a teacher from Durgapur who has conceived in her forties with donor eggs, talks about her deepest fears:

> Abhi humne apne kids ko kuch bola nahi hai that they are born out of egg donor [We haven't told our kids that they are born out of egg donor]. We might tell them or we might not tell them, depending upon the situation. I spoke to someone who told me that there is no need of telling. It is okay. If there is someone else's blood in your body that doesn't mean that your body becomes someone else's. So, wahi yahan pe bhi hai [that's exactly the same case]. But then I have seen my husband and my mother-in-law the way they behave with me and my kids, slyly hinting that she is not your proper mum.[56]

The biggest problem with donor IVF is your mind. I have seen so many couples who are stuck in the phase of self IVF even when the doctor has indicated that their chances are slim in this process. One after the other IVF fails and they keep changing doctors, looking for someone who will help them conceive through self IVF. What they don't understand is that doctors are ultimately human, and they can't push you towards something for which you are not prepared. Also, IVF is a game of chances—you might

---

56 Interview with Sumita, a teacher, Durgapur.

conceive with self IVF, but then the chances are lesser when compared to donor IVF.

On the other hand, as donor cycles are more expensive than self and chances of success are more, doctors prefer donor cycles, and in some cases, clinics are known to push you towards the donor cycle even if you might not need it at that point of time.

Now, this is a very difficult situation and decision. Only you can decide because ultimately doctors will swing the way you want to.

Remember, a donor cycle has no legal, ethical or moral obligation. It is not adoption. You don't have to sign any papers or tell anyone—not even the kid born out of it—and no donor is coming to blackmail you as seen in Bollywood movies.

YOUR MOTHERHOOD IS NOT JUST AN EGG

Guys, it is just an egg.

The baby grows in your body, receives your blood stream and nutrition, reads your thoughts. And most importantly, the baby comes out of you after nine months, unlike in surrogacy where you are not pregnant, and then justifying having a baby after nine months is an issue.

It is just an egg that you waste every month. Even if the egg is not yours, the body in which the embryo grows is yours. The baby grows inside you, so you don't need to explain anything to anyone. It is just a couple's decision and should remain between them only. Don't make it an ethical issue and spoil your chance of conception. If your medical background clearly indicates towards donor cycle, it is best not to waste any more time. In IVF, age is critical. Below thirty-five years, IVF success rate is higher comparatively. Pregnancy rate with embryo donor cycle is a 60–70 per cent per attempt.

As hard as it might seem, try to keep your emotions at bay. Scrutinize your case like a detective. Then weigh in all your options and take an informed and practical decision. There is no point going for round after round of IVF, burning away money and spoiling your health and wellbeing just because you are fixated on conceiving through your own egg or sperm.

I know it is a tough decision. Here are few things you can do in the process of reaching the right decision:

- Get a second opinion. Check with two to three doctors and get a consensus. You might waste consultation charges, but then it is better than a failed cycle. However, the problem is every doctor will ask you to get some tests done before they give their opinion. So, in such a case, I would tell the doctor straight up that I am here to get your opinion, and if what you say makes logical sense to me, I might think of changing my current doctor. Trust me! This worked like magic every time.
- Scrutinize your medical situation, your mental state, and all other factors minutely. Then solve your own mystery because no one knows your body or mind better than you.

- Trust your gut feeling. A word of caution here—don't take decision if you are stressed or feeling frustrated, anxious or angry.
- Take advice from someone who has already been through the journey like a fertility counsellor or meet a psychologist.

Fresh and Frozen IVF Cycle

Fresh IVF cycle means that eggs retrieved in that cycle are used for that cycle itself. Whereas in a frozen IVF cycle, the aim is to give a stimulant to get maximum eggs, and then use some in the current IVF cycle while saving some for the next cycle(s) by freezing them. You save on cost and a repeat of the pain and discomfort of the initial two steps of stimulation and egg retrieval. By this method, you can go for more number of IVFs than what your body can normally bear.

I don't advise more than three IVFs if the complete protocol is followed. However, with frozen IVF cycle, you have a few more chances, depending on your medical history and financial capacity. I know a couple who conceived on their eleventh frozen cycle IVF. Still, based on my personal experience, I would cap it at maximum four to five frozen IVF cycles.

Also, don't be misled when someone says that they conceived after eight IVF cycles. Please ask them if there were fresh or frozen cycles. Don't be naively mislead into believing that you can do round after round of IVF. Trust me, your body, and most importantly, your mind will give up after three cycles. That should be a cue for you to look beyond IVF.

Another debate regarding fresh vs frozen IVF cycles is with regard to success probabilities. Some doctors strongly believe that fresh IVF cycles have better chances of success as the freezing and thawing process impact the egg quality. Some eggs get wasted during the thawing process. On the other hand, another set of doctors will say that when you do fresh cycle transfer, it takes a toll on your body, as embryo transfer is done after three or five days of egg retrieval (a minor surgical intervention done under anaesthesia). Planning a frozen cycle after a month or two gives the body time to recuperate and also focus on getting the endometrium lining and hormone levels absolutely conducive for embryo transfer.

Clearly, this is a non-conclusive debate where you have to take a decision based on multiple factors like how many eggs were retrieved, your age, your financial capacity (each frozen IVF cycle is an added cost, but the cost is lesser than a full fresh IVF cycle) and medical reasons (like thin or unresponsive endometrium lining or a case of ovarian hyper-stimulation). Take an informed decision.

Breaking Up the Costs

While IVF is a blessing in disguise for couples dealing with infertility, the IVF cost is something which can pose serious financial troubles.

If you and your spouse are considering IVF treatments in India, one of the first things that you should be cognizant of is the charges for IVF treatment. In fact, you should plan and prepare for it in advance.

Generally, the charges for IVF treatment in India is anywhere between Rs 60,000 and Rs 80,000, inclusive of medicines. However, in reality, most couples end up spending more than Rs 5 lakhs on IVF treatment and procedures due to the need for several rounds of IVF cycles.

Abhiroop, thirty-four years old, software engineer from Hyderabad says, 'If a clinic quotes you 2 lakhs for the IVF process, in my experience you need to be prepared for atleast double the amount factoring in any hysteroscopy, uterus scratching or any other procedure that might need to be done.'[57]

If you are looking for affordable IVF options in India, you will need to take all these factors into consideration.

Table 6.1: IVF Treatment Costs in India

Assisted IVF with Egg Donor	Rs 2,50,000
Embryo Donor	Rs 55,000
Frozen Embryos Transfer	Rs 30,000
Testicular Sperm Aspiration	Rs 18,000
Intracytoplasmic Sperm Injection	Rs 2,20,000

Note: All the costs shown in this table are indicative and might change based on location and medical history.
Source: Created by the author.

---

[57] Interview with Abhiroop, a thirty-four-year-old software engineer, Hyderabad.

Cost of Sperm Donor IVF

Couples with low or bad quality sperms/eggs may require a donor. The cost of the sperm donor varies between Rs 8,000 and Rs 12,000 in India.

Cost of Assisted IVF with Egg Donor

An assisted IVF cycle with egg donor is a bit tricky and expensive. The cost of donor eggs can vary between Rs 50,000 and Rs 80,000, depending on the qualification of a donor. This is an added cost to regular IVF.

> Total cost of egg donor IVF cycle is:
> Rs 50,000 + Rs 2,00,000 = Rs 2,50,000 lakhs (approximately)
> (Cost of donor eggs) + (Cost of IVF cycle)

Note: A certain portion of the IVF treatment cost, which is usually Rs 30,000, is paid to the woman who is providing her eggs, while a certain percentage is given to the agent or the agency that arranges for it. Though it is not legal, this is how it works. The New ART Bill has brought major changes to the donor IVF process, which ensures that the donor (usually poor women) rights, payment and safety protocols are strictly followed.

Cost of Embryo Donor for IVF

Many a times, fertility specialists suggest embryo donors if either one or both the partners have serious genetic health conditions that can be inherited by their kids. In such cases, doctors use embryos of fertile people with no serious medical history. The cost of embryos donor for IVF can range between Rs 35,000 and Rs 55,000. With the recent ART bill and some major changes in donor IVF protocols. With the recent ART bill and some major changes in donor IVF protocols, donor IVF cost is set to increase.

Cost of Frozen Embryos Transfer for IVF

Nowadays, many couples prefer to freeze their embryos through an IVF procedure so that they can be transferred to the woman's uterus later. In India, the cost of frozen embryo transfer can vary between Rs 20,000 and Rs 30,000, excluding the cost of surrogacy.

Cost of Testicular Sperm Aspiration for IVF

Sperm aspiration and extraction procedure is prescribed for men who go for vasectomy. It is a minor procedure in which sperm is extracted directly from the testicle through a needle. The cost of testicular sperm aspiration can vary anywhere between Rs 12,000 and Rs 18,000.

Cost of ICSI for IVF

An ICSI procedure is used when a male partner has infertility issues like low or poor sperm count. A doctor injects a single sperm directly into a woman's body to fertilize the egg. This procedure can cost anywhere between Rs 20,000 and Rs 45,000. This is an added cost to the regular IVF treatment cost.

Total cost of ICSI is:

Rs 20,000 + Rs 2,00,000 = Rs 2,20,000 lakhs (approximately)
(Cost of ICSI) + (Cost of IVF cycle)

IVF Treatment Cost for International Patients in India

Considering the fact that IVF treatment cost is lower in India as compared to the rest of the world, many international infertile patients also visit the country for this treatment. Here is the IVF treatment cost that foreign couples would have to bear in India:

1. $2500 for normal IVF with your eggs and sperms.
2. $4500 for assisted IVF cycle which requires egg donor.

However, Veera Karthik originally from Bengaluru and currently residing in Australia shares with disgrunt, 'A different bracket applies to you if you come from overseas. Even though you are Indian citizens, you get charged rates like NRIs.'

Well! That's the sad reality and we can't do much about it as of now.

Cost of Preimplantation Genetic Diagnosis (PGD)

PGD or preimplantation genetic screening (PGS) is a technique to test embryos for any genetic medical condition so that only healthy embryos are placed into a woman's uterus. It is a useful step for couples who have genetic disorders but don't want it to pass on to their child. Usually, it costs above Rs 5,000 per embryo.

Mild Versus Aggressive IVF Treatment Price

Usually, mild IVF is done in case of the first IVF cycle, which can cost you Rs 1.5 lakhs approximately. In the case of aggressive IVF treatment, the cost of IVF can range from Rs 1.75 to 2 lakhs. The primary difference between both these IVF treatments lies in the dosage of medicines and injections. Gonal injections are usually very expensive.

Cost of Important Tests

Before initiating IVF or IUI, the doctor will conduct some diagnostic and corrective tests, which are both crucial and expensive. They are:

1. **Laparoscopy** (diagnostic and corrective): It is required for endometriosis patients, and it can cost anywhere between Rs 50,000 and Rs 70,000.
2. **HSG**: It is done to check the fertility potential in a female and can cost anywhere between Rs 5,000 and Rs 8,000.

IVF treatment cost in Government Hospitals

Government hospitals in India also offer IVF treatment at a much cheaper cost.

However, government hospitals might be crowded, doctors might be a bit unfriendly (due to managing large volumes), the system more time-consuming, but the quality of treatment is good as the doctors are quite experienced. They can do a normal IVF from Rs 70,000 to 1 lakh (inclusive of all the tests, etc.).

Cost of Freezing Embryos

Nowadays, many career-oriented women are planning ahead and opting to freeze their embryos so that they can be used later. The cost of freezing embryos involves the initial cost of the procedure along with annual charges which are levied to secure the frozen eggs. The initial cost of extracting eggs can go up to Rs 30,000 with annual charges of Rs 4,000–6,000 to preserve them.

Factors Which Influence the Total IVF Treatment Cost in India

Location

IVF treatment cost in India majorly depends on your location. Thus, IVF treatment cost in Mumbai is much higher than in Meerut. Due to these huge differences in cost, many couples prefer to travel to other cities in search of affordable IVF in India.

Here's an indicative price list of IVF treatments in different India states:

Table 6.2: Average Cost Per IVF Treatment Cycle in Indian Rupees (Not Inclusive of Medicines and Blood Tests)

Mumbai	2,00,000–3,00,000
Bangalore	1,60,000–1,75,000
Chennai	1,45,000–1,60,000
Delhi	90,000–1,25,000
Nagpur	75,000–90,000
Hyderabad	70,000–90,000
Pune	65,000–85,000

Source: Created by the author.

Woman's Age

Usually, a woman under thirty-five has more chances of getting pregnant with her first IVF cycle. Those above thirty-five may require three or more IVF cycles to conceive. More the number of IVF cycles needed means higher the treatment cost.

So do factor in your age while planning out your IVF treatment budget to avoid the financial and emotional stress of unexpected rounds of treatment. Each IVF cycle is important as we never want to go for another cycle. No one wants their IVF cycle to fail, and for this, you must avoid the mistakes (discussed in details in Chapter 7) and prepare well through proper research, make informed decisions, have a prepared approach and proactiveness.

Further, there are some infertility clinics in India which offer IVF plans with multiple cycle processes. This can work out better for older couples who have a tight budget.

Remember, even though the charges for IVF treatment in India varies from one city to another, you should never choose a clinic merely on the basis of cost. Always look for a fertility specialist who has a good reputation with a high success rate.

Stay Away from Marketing Gimmicks

You should know that the IVF market is highly competitive. Setting and running an IVF clinic is expensive as it is an advanced treatment. One cycle of IVF costs Rs 1–2.5 lakhs approximately. Add to it the cost of multiple tests. A couple who has not been able to conceive for a few years is desperate, and this desperation leads to doctor-shopping. You want to find the best IVF doctor as the costs of an IVF cycle is high, and so is your hope. This attitude of couples leads to a stiff competition between the IVF clinics who often employ aggressive marketing gimmicks to lure in couples.

Stay away from:

1. **False claims:** You will come across some clinics who will claim 90% IVF success rates or guaranteed pregnancy to lure you in. Please ask for concrete and documented proof of their claims over an email sent from their official email id or signed on their letterhead,

if they hesitate (which they will) then you know what to do.

2. **Bundle packages**: They ask you to pay for three IVF cycles together at a discounted price at the onset itself. No matter how practical it sounds, I don't agree with this arrangement. I would give my best to the first IVF cycle itself and want it to be successful. So, if I choose this arrangement, I will end up paying way too much. In another scenario, if I wait till the third IVF with the same doctor, I will end up causing much damage to my body (invasive processes, heavy medications, surgical processes do have side effects), not to mention the mental agony of repeated failed IVFs.

3. **Cashback schemes**: In this instance, some clinics tell you to pay for IVF, and if it doesn't succeed, they will give you some cashback. Again, I don't agree with this on ethical grounds. Anything that starts with a proposition of failure can't be a good start.

4. **Hideous Clinic Protocols**: One of the biggest challenges for the couples seeking IVF is the lack of transparency in the cost by the clinics. The hidden costs of last-minute scans or tests increase the cost significantly. Some clinics will quote a certain amount at the time of registration as package cost and later would give an inflated bill quoting exclusions which the patient was neither clearly informed or asked for consent. If you are going for a package deal ask about all exclusions clearly.

How Can You Save Money?

EMI-Free Loan Option

You can pay by credit card and then keep paying back with 0 per cent interest. Some IVF clinics in collaboration with third party financing agencies provide these facilities. Always ask your clinic about cost management options that are available. Companies like LetsMD, Tata Capital, MoneyTap, BankBazaar, PaisaBazaar, Bajaj Finserv are some of the places where you can get unsecured medical loans. Or, if you have good credit limit, pay by credit card. The good thing about these loans is that you can get them quickly with least documentation but remember to negotiate hard (they might have hidden charges) and choose the one that is the right fit for you.

Buy Injections and Medicine from Wholesale Pharmacies

In the IVF process, it is the injections that eat up the maximum cost. However, wholesale pharmacies provide these injections and medicines at a much cheaper cost, thus saving you a lot of money. Obviously, you'll have to put in extra effort by looking them up, travelling to a certain point, etc. Also, do check with your clinic first. Many clinics insist that you buy the full package (treatment, diagnostic test, medicines and injection—all costs included) and will give you some random theory, not allowing you to get medicines/injections from pharmacy/diagnostic test from outside their clinic. However, you are not bound to them legally, so speak sternly if need be.

Public Trust and Government Hospitals

In a bid to curtail the cost of infertility treatment and make it accessible, the public trust Nowrosjee Wadia Maternity Hospital in Mumbai opened a new IVF centre (in 2016) called the Wadia Assisted Reproduction Technology Centre. Inaugurated by the then Maharashtra Health Minister, Deepak Sawant, it is the first public trust hospital opened in the state where IVF treatment is done at half the rates.

You can find similar trusts and government-run hospitals in India. In Delhi, the All India Institute of Medical Sciences (AIIMS) and Safdarjung Hospital run low-cost IVF programmes. In West Bengal, the Institute of Post Graduate Medical Education and Research is the first government hospital to provide fertility treatments at accessible costs. There are also many private clinics that provide discounts if the patient can prove that they belong to a lower income group.

Personal Insurance for Infertility Treatment

Sadly, while maternity is covered by all insurance schemes in India, infertility/ART/IVF treatment isn't a favourite with providers offering personal insurance. Even if some insurance providers (Star Health Insurance and New India Insurance) do have a policy coverage for infertility, there might be some restrictive criteria of the claim like waiting period (coverage benefit can be availed only after a certain number of years of buying the policy) or eligibility (just covering a certain part of the treatment/diagnostic process) or validity (you can avail the benefit for only one IVF cycle) or a pre-existing condition (you should not have infertility while buying the policy or you haven't disclosed at the time of policy purchase). Read the fine print carefully. Generally, infertility treatment coverage insurance is expensive.

Corporate/Office Insurance

If you or your partner is working in a corporate company then you might be covered under corporate group insurance if not for IVF treatment then for follow-up surgeries like hysteroscopy, egg freezing or a laparoscopy. Make sure to check with your company HR on the coverage.

Arshi Khazir, a thirty-five-year-old analyst who works in Accenture, Mumbai was very happy as her company has this facility for their employees called Vidal health which covers IVF under fertility treatments to the extent of Rs 1 Lakhs. She claimed and got Rs 90,000 against IVF treatment covering atleast half of her expense on the treatment. She also adds,

> Accenture has very good policies in terms of leaves and insurance. They provide adoption, surrogacy, miscarriage leaves separately. And even they understand about your issues. I asked my senior

manager to give me project where there is less work pressure because I am going through IVF treatment, they agreed and told me not to worry and to focus on my treatment. So, touch wood, being with Accenture and having WFH I am managing these fertility treatments.

You will be required to upload all your treatment prescriptions, bills and lab reports to claim the insurance. Make a habit of stacking it all in a folder organized as per dates. Trust me! You will thank me for this tip. Every time, I would go for my consultation and the doctor would ask for my last report, I would have all the papers strewn on the desk and would never find the right one at the right time. Well! Technology has been a boon now so you can even maintain all your health records digitally for easy access and automatic organization.

If you are working in public sector companies or a government office some treatment coverage is available though there might be some documentation like the hospital you are planning for treatment should be empaneled with them and you might be required to submit documentary proof from the gynecologist that you need an IVF. They might have some restrictions on age (especially if you are above 40 years, they might reject your claim) or number of IUI/IVF attempts. The coverage might be capped. The good thing is to check with your company and get as much financial support as you can so that you can focus more on preparing for the treatment.

Financing Schemes

Most IVF clinics have some sort of basic financing through credit card, where you can pay money in parts. However, be mindful since the interest rates might be on the higher side. There are many apps and even banks that provide facilities of EMI or the 'Pay Later' option.

Personal Loan

You can also take a personal loan to finance your treatment cost. As a personal loan can be used for any purpose, it is of great help for couples planning for IVF but are constrained by money. Recently, many apps have been launched that provide short term personal loans.

Research and Referral Institutes, Defence Forces

If you are connected with the Army, Air Force, or Navy you can avail benefits of specialized Artificial Reproductive Technology (ART) centres in army hospitals located at Delhi, Pune, Mumbai, Bhopal, etc. In these centres, the treatment is free of cost. However, there are some criteria that one should fulfil to avail the benefit. For people working in Border Roads or other allied defence services there are options to reimburse treatment cost through CGHS (Central Government Health Insurance Scheme) or Ex-servicemen Contributory Health Scheme (ECHS). The reimbursable amount differs from organization to organization. Connect with your medical officer for more information.

Where Should You NOT Save Money?

Once you have decided on the IVF path, there are some aspects where you should not be penny wise pound foolish.

Don't be Too Price Sensitive

You must research well before deciding on an IVF clinic. Visit and talk to multiple clinics and ask questions. However, don't make price the only consideration. Also, do not compare notes with what another couple undergoing fertility treatment is paying. I can't tell you how many couples come to me every day and say, 'They just paid Rs 1 lakh for IVF treatment and my clinic is asking me to pay more.'

It is important to understand that IVF is usually tailored to your specific needs. There can be many variations of IVF and with each new twist or test, the cost varies.

The cost of IVF is an important aspect, but it should not be the sole deciding factor. Do take into consideration all the factors before choosing a clinic that is the right fit for you.

Preparation

For IVF to be successful preparation of the body and mind are equally important. It is important that your body is in its best shape for IVF to work efficiently. Holistic approaches that include alternative therapies are a good way to prepare yourself for this excruciatingly intensive treatment. When you are already paying Rs 1–2.5 lakhs for IVF, spend a little more and prepare yourself well.

Natural treatments like Ayurveda have excellent results in detoxing and building your internal immunity. Ayurveda also works well to improve sperm quality.

Declutter your mind and learn to manage anxiety because it is bound to happen. You may seek the help of an expert or opt for guided meditation sessions. Take up some physical activity like yoga or a sport.

Though there is no recorded research, there have been amazing results of employing acupuncture in IVF conception if done before the embryo transfer stage.

Work on your relationship goals. Go on vacation before starting IVF.

We will discuss more about alternative methodologies and its impact in Chapter 7.

For now, it is about setting the right mindset and focusing. Prepare yourself well.

A Roadmap to Plan Better

Having a roadmap will help you manage financial stress so that you can immerse yourself in the treatment with a positive mindset. Even if in your case managing finance is the male partner's primary responsibility, he can't simply stay detached from the IVF process by saying, 'She (wife) will get the IVF done and I (husband) will manage the finances.' As a husband, you must be involved in every step of the process as IVF is a physically and mentally strenuous process. The stress, if not managed properly, will creep in and impact the treatment because ultimately both you and your partner are one unit.

Sit, talk and discuss every detail. In fact, you should draw up a roadmap before going for your first IVF. Run through the possibilities like:

1. How many IVF cycles can you afford?
2. Always have a Plan B: Don't pin all your hopes on one IVF cycle or on one mode of financial planning. Diversify and have a Plan B.
3. Don't take loans.

I met a couple who said that they would sell off their property and go to any length to treat infertility. I paused, looked in their eyes and asked, 'What kind of life would you give the baby?'

You need to understand why you want a baby in the first place. Is it some kind of race where you have to reach an elusive finish line? Or is it based in ego?

Think hard, think calmly.

7

The Different Types of IVF and their Step-by-Step Process

My first IVF failed primarily because I was constantly thinking about what would happen next, which increased my anxiety to another level.

IN THIS CHAPTER, I WILL TRY TO EXPLAIN THE IVF PROCESS IN an easy manner so that you know what to expect and are able to navigate the IVF journey with confidence. It is also important to understand the medical jargon so that you are not intimidated and you can make an informed decision. You have to take many decisions during the IVF process and knowing the answers in advance is just good housekeeping.

Preparation Pointers:

1. Self-knowledge of the subject.
2. Complete understanding of your medical case.

3. Understand what the doctor says.
4. Assess your goals.

Once you have a deep understanding of the above points, it'll help you make the right treatment-related decision. Just remember that what works for someone else won't work for you. You may develop insights by talking to other people and listening to their stories, but finally, you have to take into consideration the above factors and create your own magic formula.

At this stage, you should also ask your doctor the right questions.

'Women are expressive, and at every consultation, they will show their desperation. This becomes repetitive to the point of irritation. In fact, it is not easy to answer questions than constantly require reassurance that I can set everything right. This becomes challenging,' says Dr Parul Katiyar, senior IVF specialist, New Delhi.

Doctors are not God. They are doing their best in the given situation. They can answer your questions logically and follow protocol. So, try to rein in overtly emotional responses.

The Step-by-Step Process of IVF

Step 1: Pre-Preparation

Some IVF protocols require you to take birth control pills one cycle prior to the IVF cycle. For example, say you have to undergo IVF in March; in that case, some doctors will put you on birth control pills from January or February. These are prescribed if:

1. You have a cyst that needs to be shrunk.
2. You are going for batch IVF where the menstrual cycles of a group of women are synced with the help of medications in such a way that they ovulate almost around the same time, thus making it easier for doctors to conduct the egg retrieval process of a batch of women on the same day.
3. To time your period cycle better.

Step 2: Growth of Follicles — The Stimulation Phase

Day 1 of the menstrual cycle is considered to be the starting point of the IVF cycle. Doctors usually ask you to call on day 1 or day 2 of the menstrual cycle to schedule an appointment for blood tests, ultrasound and pre-IVF checkups. The pelvic (or vaginal) ultrasound is done between three and five days to evaluate the ovaries, and a blood test is done to check the hormone levels. If all is okay, then you are scheduled to start on FSH hormone injections that stimulate the growth of egg follicles. This phase will take eight to twelve days, depending on the growth of your follicles and your body's response to stimulus medicines. Be prepared to take injections, medicines, and go for ultrasound tests; overall, it is not a pleasant experience.

Table 7.1: Stages of the IVF Process

Day 1	Menstrual cycle/periods start.
Day 1/Day 2	Inform the doctor and book an appointment for the tests.
Day 3–5	Get pre-IVF workup tests done.
Day 12 onwards	Hormone/Progesterone Injections start.
Day 14–16	Trigger injection given on the day when the eggs are just ready to ovulate and when the eggs are retrieved.
Day 17–22	Embryos are made and then transferred on day 3 or day 5 of the retrieval or frozen to be transferred next month or later (as the case maybe).
Day 36–38	Fourteen days after the embryo transfer, the pregnancy blood test is done to confirm the implantation.

Note: This table is indicative and there might be slight change depending on your IVF protocol and period cycle.

Source: Created by the author.

Blood tests and ultrasound are repeated several times during a cycle to measure follicle growth and check hormone levels, so that the dosage of FSH can be increased or decreased accordingly. You might have to visit the clinic every day or every alternate day to receive injections and do ultrasounds to follow the growth of follicles.

The whole purpose of this process is to control the timing of the egg ripening, thus increasing the chances of having multiple eggs. Although more eggs are good, more than 15–20 along with high oestriodal counts increases the chances of a complication called Ovarian Hyper-Stimulation Syndrome (OHSS).[58]

During this phase, you may feel a sense of heaviness and bloating as your ovaries are producing more than the normal number of follicles. It might be a little discomforting. It is better to take it easy during this phase and not do heavy tasks.

Step 3: Release of Eggs

Once the follicles have reached a certain size and are ready to be released, a trigger injection of HCG is administered, which allows the eggs to undergo a final step of maturation. Timing is critical here. Usually, egg collection is scheduled thirty-six to thirty-eight hours after the trigger injection. For this step, you need to be at the clinic when required.

Step 4: Egg Retrieval

To retrieve the eggs, the doctor inserts an ultrasound probe into the vagina, and then, with the help of a needle, withdraws the eggs from the follicles. The patient is under

---

[58] M.M. Alper, L.P. Smith and F.S. Sills, 'Ovarian Hyperstimulation Syndrome: Current Views on Pathophysiology, Risk Factors, Prevention, and Management', *Journal of Experimental and Clinical Assisted Reproduction* 6, no. 3 (2009), available at https://www.ncbi.nlm.nih.gov/pmc/articles/PMC2868304/.

sedation during this procedure, which takes approximately fifteen to thirty minutes, depending on the number of follicles present. You may experience light bleeding, vaginal discharge and pelvic cramps. These are normal symptoms unless they become severe, in which case you should check with your doctor. You will be monitored for a couple of hours and asked to return home and rest for the day.

At the same time, your partner is asked to give a sperm sample.

Step 5: Embryo-Making in the Lab

This is one of the most important stages of IVF because this is literally where the lab will develop your baby in a test tube.

The embryologist will begin the procedure of embryo development in the lab. The various stages of this process are:

1. Retrieved eggs move towards maturity under close monitoring.
2. Sperm are introduced to mature eggs for fertilization.
3. Fertilization checks are conducted to sieve out abnormal embryos.
4. Embryos begin to multiply as cells on day three, when there are about six to eight cells.
5. The embryo is transferred on day three (the embryo is three days old) or on day five (the blastocyst stage where the embryo is five days old), depending on the type of IVF protocol you have chosen.

Usually, embryos formed may be fewer than the eggs retrieved. This happens when:

1. Not all eggs are mature.
2. Those eggs that mature may form abnormal embryos on fertilization.
3. Normal embryos may not reach up to day three.
4. And day three embryos might stop growing on day five.

As you can see, there are many challenges before the perfect embryo reaches the next stage of transfer.

Step 6: Embryo Transfer

On day three or day five, the embryo is transferred. It never happens on day four. If any clinic schedules a transfer on day four, you need to stay alert and ask them why it's being done. Day four is called the morula stage—a dynamic day when embryos show no movement at all, making it difficult to ascertain their status. No decision should be made on this day.

In a normal IVF, it's usually on day three that the embryo transfer is scheduled. For couples with a history of failed IVF cycles, mostly owing to implantation issue, day five, also known as the blastocyst stage, is advised. The benefits of the blastocyst stage transfer, in simple terms, are:

1. Surer in this game of probability.
2. On day five, the embryo outgrows the outer shell, breaks from it, and is ready to implant. Thus, this

timing increases the chances of implantation and IVF success.
3. The embryos that don't move to the blastocyst stage are discarded, further reducing the chances of an abnormal embryo.
4. Couples who opt for genetic testing (like PGS or PGD) have to wait till the blastocyst stage in order to facilitate the process.

When the embryo is transferred on day three, it keeps floating in the uterus until it reaches the blastocyst stage and then implants.

However, the problem with blastocyst transfer is that this is an advanced technique, and your clinic's lab should be equipped with both the equipment and a full-time embryologist to do it justice. Also, it is an added cost.

The embryo transfer process is the same on both days three and five. One or more of the fertilized embryos are placed in the uterus with the help of a thin, flexible catheter, inserted through the cervix.

You are asked to keep your bladder full, which makes it easy for the doctor to examine the uterus properly, thus facilitating the embryos to land as close to the uterus as possible. On the flip side, keeping your bladder full is tricky. A lady once told me that she couldn't hold it any longer and peed in the last minute, exactly when the embryo was taken into the vial. She, therefore, wasted her cycle and money. In another incident, a woman drank excess water, and as a result, the doctor couldn't see her uterus properly. The doctor had to take out the excess water through a catheter in the OT before doing the transfer.

An anxious mind, a full bladder, and the scary OT is not really an ideal combo. You must have a full bladder and get into OT for the process. So, you can't alter these two but what you can control is your anxiety and that can change the results for you. That's why I can't emphasize enough on the importance of learning to manage anxiety.

Embryo transfer is done without anaesthesia. A maximum of two to three embryos are transferred, but ideally, it should be one per cycle. The extra embryos can either be frozen for the next cycle or discarded. You will have to take a call on that. However, doctors can't transfer more embryos even if you made a good batch. It is important to ensure that there is a full-term and healthy pregnancy that follows. IVF still births and twin child complications are quite common.

Box 7.1: An Important Tip from Personal Experience

> To maximize the success of an embryo transfer, try to hold still after the procedure. The nurse will want to move you from the OT stretcher to a normal bed. See if you can avoid that. Hold your pee for as long as possible. Control your mind to be balanced. Imagery meditation techniques can help. Focus on your breathing. Think of good and happy things.

Source: Created by the author.

Step 7: The Two-Week Waiting Period

After the transfer, you need to rest for at least seventy-two hours. It is in these first three to four days after the embryo transfer that the implantation happens.

When I asked women undergoing infertility treatments (women who are part of my Fertility Dost infertility support group) what the most difficult part of their journey was, most of them said that it was the anxiety of the waiting period.

When you go through a particular infertility treatment that promises conception, you are extremely anxious till the result comes out. In the case of IVF, this usually takes two weeks.

It is the failure behind the wait that we fear the most. It is latching onto the last bit of hope that keeps us anxious.

'On the fourteenth day after the transfer, I was tense whether the report would be positive or not. It's like waiting for the results of a final exam, with that constant feeling of whether you passed or failed. I will never forget how fast my heart was beating on the beta HCG test (blood test to confirm pregnancy) day', says Shveta, thirty-five-year-old homemaker from Gurugram.

'The two weeks' wait period is definitely the worst part! Even in my deepest sleep, I used to worry. I surfed the internet so much because I didn't have much to do. Not to mention, facing your beta HCG result, the persistent thought of what next in case of failure never left me', says

Arti (thirty-two years old) and Dinesh (thirty-six years old), a couple from Gwalior who are currently in Dubai, working with a construction company.

After the embryo transfer, I used to play every teenager's favourite game of 'he loves me, he loves me not', but with a twist; 'Will I be pregnant? Or not?'

There are no guarantees. This period of fifteen to twenty days is all about luck, God's will, the preparation you have done before, and the decisions you have taken. Medical science, although extremely advanced, has no role to play here. And this ambiguity is what causes fear, and fear breeds anxiety.

Managing Your Thoughts

'It felt lonely. That is a fact of life. People can be with you, but they can't take injections for you', said Sukhpreet, a twenty-nine-year-old interior designer from Chandigarh, whose thoughts will resonate with anyone going through the treatment.

Anxiety is natural at this stage but try to not allow it to take over you. It's only natural to have negative thoughts, but you need to observe them without getting flustered by them. They are only thoughts, after all, and will soon pass. However, you can realign your negative thoughts. For example, if you had a failed IVF cycle earlier, when thoughts such as, 'It failed last time, what will happen now?' arise, try telling yourself, 'It failed last time because of XYZ reason, but this time, I chose to rectify that and did better, so my chances will be better. But if the IVF fails this time as well, I will follow my Plan B,'

In Chapter 8, we talk about the plan. In anxious moments like these, a Plan B can take the pressure off the present situation. I myself did this and it worked to ease my anxiety.

Step 8: Pregnancy Confirmation Test

Two weeks after the embryo transfer, a blood urine test is done to determine HCG levels. This hormone confirms pregnancy. If the first HCG level is <5 IU/L, the pregnancy is negative; if the level is >10 IU/L, the test is repeated every forty-eight hours to confirm that the levels are doubling. The levels should double every forty-eight hours in the first twenty-one days after the embryo transfer. If the second HCG levels do not increase, the test is repeated after forty-eight hours. Even then if it does not increase, then chances are that the pregnancy is not progressing.

If HCG levels increase, a pelvic ultrasound is done after three to four weeks to make sure the gestational sac is visible. A heartbeat can be heard after about six to six-and-a-half weeks of pregnancy, which is approximately four to four-and-a-half weeks post transfer.

Donor Egg IVF Cycle

In donor IVF, the process remains the same with regard to the different tasks for different people. There are two parties involved in this process, namely the donor and the recipient. The couple who wants to have the baby and will bear the embryo in the (female partner's) uterus is called the recipient, and the woman who provides egg for making the embryo is called the donor.

Choosing the right donor is an important task. However, when it comes to choosing the donor, most couples are so obsessed with getting the physical features right that they overlook the medical parameters. Ensure that all tests of the donor lady are done properly and the doctor selects the donor after a thorough medical check. These medical tests, especially the hormone markers, should be assessed and reassessed over a period of three to six months as hormone markers do change from month to month. Genetic tests are important to ensure that no genetic abnormality is passed onto the baby through the donor.

Donors are usually younger women who already have a child.

The stimulation and egg retrieval phases are done on the donor. The sperm is provided by the recipient partner, and the embryo transfer process is done on the recipient lady.

Table 7.2: Steps in the Donor Egg IVF Cycle

Donor	Recipient
Step 1: Pre-Preparation	Step 5: Embryo-Making in the Lab
Step 2: Growth of Follicles—The Stimulation Phase	Step 6: Embryo Transfer

Donor	Recipient
Step 3: Release of Eggs	Step 7: The Two-Week Waiting Period
Step 4: Egg Retrieval	Step 8: Pregnancy Confirmation Test

Source: Created by the author.

Shared Versus Exclusive Donor

This is another concept that you should be aware of, where you can choose to have an exclusive donor to yourself or share her eggs with others. Normally, a donor produces somewhere between twenty plus eggs.

Under the shared donor concept, the clinic ensures that you get enough eggs for at least two IVF cycles. The remaining eggs are shared with another recipient. The cost of these donor eggs, ranging from Rs 40,000–50,000 is almost half of the exclusive one.

In the exclusive donor arrangement, as the name suggests, all the eggs of the donor are at your disposal. However, the cost will be around Rs 70,000–80,000, in addition to the regular IVF cost. Otherwise, the process is absolutely the same. It is just a matter of personal choice and ethics.

The donor and the recipient's cycles are synced. While the donor is prepared for egg formation, the recipient *prepares her endometrial lining for implantation* (it should be at least 7 millimetres). The recipient woman will also be taking medicines and injections, though much fewer than those taken in a self-egg IVF cycle.

As a recipient woman, you need to prepare your mind and body well to increase your IVF success rates. Moreover, it is in you that the baby grows, so *you* are the single-most important person right now.

A few points:

1. Take *folic acid* for at least three months before the transfer of embryos.
2. Start on a *healthy diet* of vitamins and minerals.
3. Keep your *mind strong* and your body fit.
4. *Exercise.*
5. Try *alternative treatment* methodologies to increase your endometrium lining and immunity.

What Can Go Wrong During IVF?

In this section, we focus on things that can go wrong during the IVF process due to which the cycle stands cancelled or postponed. Keep an eye out for these instances. Though they are not common occurrences, they can completely ruin your IVF cycle and also lead to a waste of money.

Doctors usually avoid mentioning these possible risks, but as a patient, you have all the right to know and be mentally prepared for what you are getting into. Remember, this is meant only to educate and not to overwhelm you. And these are only *possible* risks. Mostly, you will undergo IVF without any complication at all.

Ovarian Hyper-Stimulation Syndrome (OHSS)

OHSS is a condition where your body reacts weirdly to injections given for stimulating the growth of follicles. HCG injections are quite strong and can cause pain and discomfort. For women with OHSS, it becomes quite unbearable and interferes with the IVF process.

Shreya, a thirty-two-year-old from Allahabad working in the state government, had mild PCOD, but during the stimulation phase of IVF, she had responded well. Fifteen follicles were formed and thirteen mature eggs retrieved. The night after the retrieval, she got up at midnight and threw up. She noticed that her abdomen was heavily bloated; she looked like someone who was seven or eight months pregnant. This freaked her out, so she called her doctor the next morning. She rushed to the clinic to get a scan done. The report showed that both her ovaries were swollen to 11.8 centimetres (normally, ovaries are 3–4 centimetres) in size. She had a case of extreme ovary enlargement.

Shreya was immediately admitted to the hospital and put on injections. It took three to four days for her ovaries to reduce to their normal size. But all was not okay yet. There was fluid accumulation in her lungs, which was a further cause for worry. However, she slowly recovered and was shifted to the general ward in a week. Her embryo transfer for IVF was delayed for that cycle as she had just recovered from OHSS.

Only less than 5 per cent of IVF cases in the world show OHSS syndrome, out of which only 1 per cent show severe symptoms, so you don't need to be worried but be watchful.[59]

The symptoms of OHSS are classified into four major categories, based on which action is taken; they are the following.

Mild OHSS

- Class 1: Uneasiness and discomfort in the abdominal area.
- Class 2: Both the above symptoms along with vomiting, nausea, diarrhoea and ovarian enlargement of 5–12 centimetres.

Moderate OHSS

- Class 3: All the symptoms of Classes 1 and 2 with ultrasonographic evidence of ascites (abnormal accumulation of fluid in the abdomen).

Severe OHSS

- Class 4: All the symptoms of Classes 1, 2 and 3 with breathing difficulties and/or hydrothorax (fluid accumulation in the pleural cavity).

---

59 'Ovarian Hyperstimulation Syndrome (OHSS)', Cleveland Clinic, available at https://my.clevelandclinic.org/health/diseases/17972-ovarian-hyperstimulation-syndrome-ohss.

Critical OHSS

- Class 5: All of the above symptoms, with increased blood viscosity due to hemoconcentration (blood becomes thick and concentrated), diminished renal function, change in blood volume and coagulation abnormalities.

Fluid accumulation becomes a major problem and requires aggressive management. OHSS can be managed with medicine. However, ask your doctor for low stimulation IVF protocol (low dose gonadotropin stimulation) if you are already diagnosed with OHSS. Measured and low dosage stimulation protocol with strict monitoring can successfully manage OHSS symptoms. OHSS can be managed with diet and exercise, which basically improves your body's internal immunity. Following an alkaline and non-inflammatory diet helps in such cases.

Weak Endometrium Lining

Common causes of a thin endometrium lining can be multiple miscarriages or D&Cs, suspecting or having tuberculosis or adhesions in the uterus.

Your endometrium lining is extremely important for implantation. If the lining is not well formed by the day of the embryo transfer, your embryos will be frozen, and the IVF cycle will be postponed to the next month. Women with a history of weak endometrium lining might face this issue. Eat well, as diet directly impacts your endometrium lining. You don't want to add stress by postponing the cycle in the last minute.

The good news is that there are some new ART technologies that can help improve the endometrium lining, especially if it is thin and not responding to regular treatments like medicines and diet. Ovarian platelet rich plasma (PRP) treatment is a plasma therapy where blood is collected from your body, platelet rich plasma is extracted through the centrifuge process, and then reinjected in your ovaries to regenerate the ovary and improve the endometrium lining. It is quite similar to stem cell therapy. As PRP is done using your own blood, there is no side effect.

However, it is not advised to all patients who come with thin endometrium linings. As of now, PRP treatment is at its experimental stage and is suggested to couples who have had multiple IVF failures. It is an expensive add-on to the IVF treatment, costing somewhere between Rs 10,000 and Rs 45,000, depending on what process the clinic is following, for example, whether is it injected in the body or directly into ovaries through the laparoscopy method.

Dr Rutvij Dalal, IVF doctor, Delhi, says:

> Keep your expectations modest when going for PRP treatment as it is in an experimental stage. Two leading research societies on IVF, ESHRE (European Society of Human Reproduction and Embryology) and ASRM (American Society of Reproductive Medicine) say that PRP treatment looks attractive and there are some studies but still the data isn't

enough and roughly the success rate can be placed between 10 per cent to 20 per cent.[60]

Regarding PRP treatment, remember the following:

1. Speak to your doctor clearly about the treatment.
2. Use it as a last resort or only if highly advisable in your particular case.
3. Keep moderate expectation from the treatment.
4. Ask for cost justification by clearly understanding the protocol that they are following for the PRP treatment.

Unfit Embryos

The embryologist will try to make the best embryos, but there are too many factors involved that can go wrong here:

1. Not enough eggs retrieved.
2. Eggs didn't mature.
3. Matured eggs didn't fertilize.
4. Embryos formed were not of Grade 1 or 2.
5. Embryos stopped growing.
6. Abnormal embryos.
7. Embryos didn't reach the blastocyst stage.

There are so many things that can go wrong at the embryo formation stage. This might be unnerving but IVF isn't easy.

---

60 Interview with Rutvij Dalal, IVF doctor, Delhi.

If you don't get at least one or two good embryos at the end of this process, there is no point going ahead with the IVF cycle.

Issues with the Embryology Lab

Dr Srinidhi (name changed), an MBBS doctor who herself underwent IVF, confided in me that her IVF failed because of a manual error by the embryology lab technician, and as she was being treated under her college senior, now an IVF doctor, she told her the truth, apologized, and refunded some amount of the treatment. Had she been a regular patient, do you think the doctor would have accepted the mistake? No. Instead, the doctor would have put the onus of the IVF failure on the bad quality of the embryo or would've simply said, 'We don't know what went wrong.'

The fact is that a lot can go wrong in the embryology lab. Make sure that the lab is as automated as possible, and modern technology has made it achievable. Embryoscope is one such latest technology which has a special time lapse incubator with a camera that captures embryo development in the minutest way. This facilitates the embryologist to monitor and choose the best one with perfection.

Embryos are so sensitive that even a few seconds of temperature change can finish them. An embryology lab should have an alarm system which gets triggered in case of electricity cut or a drop in temperature.

There are some artificial intelligence (AI)-driven software that can help choose the right embryo, with absolute precision precision eliminating human bias and judgement error.

Also, some clinics I know of have glass panel embryology labs and they show the couple the laboratory from outside and explain in detail about the process and technology. This really builds your trust in the clinic. After all, the embryo is your baby, and you have all the right to ensure that it is properly taken care of. It is your reproductive right.

These new-age technologies, systems and software come with an added cost; plus, only high-end clinics are currently offering these. It is good to ask the right questions and be informed. Not everyone will require these high-end tools. Worry about these tests if you have had earlier failed IVFs and that too, where the reason behind failure pointed towards bad embryo growth, irrespective of good quality eggs been retrieved.

Sperm Mixing

This is rare but does happen. Recently, a hit Bollywood movie, *Good Newwz* (2019), highlighted this issue in a humorous way. If sperm mix-up happens, it can be truly devastating for the couple. Thus, it is better to be safe than sorry and clearly ask the clinic the mechanisms they have in place to avoid sperm mixing. This situation usually doesn't happen with most good clinics who follow strict processes will either tell you at the intial stage itself or will have no problem in answering the question; however, if a clinic gives a generic/emotional answer (like 'Oh! What a silly question! Of course, we take all the precautions.') and not a technical one then you must rethink the clinic.

Ask your clinic if they use radio frequency identification (RFID) tags. Simply put, these are barcodes attached to egg and sperm samples to avoid any chances of mix-up. As eggs and sperms are microscopic, this tagging system requires advanced techniques. These labels can be read using a microscope. The more we reduce manual management, the lower are the chances of human error.

Box 7.2: Checklist to Ensure Proper Management of Embryos

1. Don't hesitate to ask your doctor about the qualification, certification and training of the embryologist.
2. Take a tour of the embryology lab.
3. Choose an IVF clinic where the embryologist is in-house and not a freelancer (an embryologist who is there only during the pick-up of the embryo and then on the transfer day, while everything in between is managed by junior technicians).
4. Speak to the embryologist.
5. Stay away from clinics who don't have dedicated embryology labs in the facility. Many clinics or different centres of the same clinic might have shared embryology labs.

Source: Created by the author.

Most Common Queries About IVF

How Much Bed Rest Should I Take?

Should I take bed rest during IVF and IUI? For how long should I take bed rest? Does bed rest means lying on the bed for the whole time, taking only loo break?

I will begin with a disclaimer that every case and treatment is different, so follow what your doctor says. However, I feel that taking bed rest is the most overrated and the biggest myth. And the type of bed rest that doesn't allow you to lay your feet on ground except loo breaks is a complete no-no. After an hour of my embryo transfer, I was lying down on the couch in the clinic's lobby, when my doctor came and asked, 'Ma'am, aren't you feeling well?'

'No, I'm fine', I said.

'Then go home, ma'am', the doctor said.

'Can I leave a little later, if it is fine by you, because I was told that I should be lying straight for the embryo to implant?' I asked.

'Ma'am, if you rest more than this, the embryo will swim out of your nose,' the doctor joked with a straight face.

Bed Rest is Overrated

You should take it slow for seventy-two hours post the embryo transfer, but beyond that there is no actual need to do so unless you have a peculiar medical condition or have been advised by your doctor. Mostly it is our parents, especially our moms and MILs, who live by the miracles of bed rest.

Trust me, most parents will emphasize on how so and so took bed rest and they became mothers.

Will you believe me if I tell you that during my first IVF cycle, I, too, like most of you, blindly followed anything and everything? I was on complete bed rest and still my IVF failed. However, in my second attempt, I resumed office after a week's break and sailed through happily. It could have been just a happy coincidence. But the failure of my first IVF cycle got me thinking about what went wrong. And one of the things that didn't work in my favour was excessive bed rest because my mind was replaying over and over, 'Will it succeed, will it not?' And this made me anxious.

Educate your parents about this aspect in a diplomatic way. Listen to your body, as you are its best judge. Don't tire yourself. Engage your mind creatively. If your mind is busy and you feel happy, your body will stay calm and composed. Paint, sing (don't dance, please), write, read, knit, go to a spa, enjoy a romantic dinner—do whatever makes you happy. Balance is the key to success.

Should I Avoid Non-Vegetarian Food During IVF?

IVF is usually the last and most complicated of infertility treatments. It takes a toll on your physical, financial and emotional wellbeing. Diet is a major concern during IVF treatment, especially the crucial period after the embryo transfer. Doctors might ask you to avoid non-vegetarian food during IVF treatment, especially foods that may increase one's body heat, popularly referred to in India as 'garam cheezein' (food items that have heat-inducing property).

When doctors ask you to avoid non-vegetarian food, they are right because during IVF you are administered with hormone injections for almost ninety days post the embryo transfer as well as before the treatment. These hormones, mainly progesterone, is known to increase body heat. Thus, it is important to not increase your body heat any further.

Seven Food Items You Must Avoid During IVF

1. **Non-vegetarian food:** You can eat fish but cooked in a light gravy. However, ensure that the fish is fresh and preferably it should be river water fresh. Avoid sea fish as it has a high mercury level and generates heat (especially if you are already taking progesterone supplements). During the IVF process, our body is injected with hormone injections which might cause metabolic issues, and thus, we don't want to add further heat to the body.
2. **Food from restaurants and outside food joints:** Don't eat food from places where you have no control the over kitchen. Stick to home-cooked food.
3. **Processed or packaged food:** Try not to pump your body with oestrogen, progesterone, testosterone, prolactin or recombinant bovine growth hormone (rBGH), especially if you are already fighting PCOD,

thyroid, diabetes, or a similar condition to make it worse, right?
4. **Absolutely no packaged juice:** They have preservatives and contain high quantities of sugar. Their nutritional value is also less, no matter how 'real' they claim to be. Make fresh juice at home. It is best to have fruits.
5. **No cold drinks:** They increase acidity due to their high sugar content for some people, so avoid any item that can disturb your bowel movements or body temperature. If you get fever (even a mild one), your IVF cycle will be cancelled.
6. **Heavy gravies or butter masala-type food:** These might lead to indigestion for some people. Due to the heavy medicines and injections you are taking during the IVF cycle, your metabolism is affected, and indigestion, acid reflux, bloating, and weight gain are the most common side effects. The ground rule is simple here—make it easy for the body to adapt to the artificial hormones injected from the outside.
7. **Raw and undercooked vegetables:** These might contain harmful bacteria that can cause infections, thus disrupting the IVF cycle. You don't want to fall sick during the process.

Infertility issues crop up due to hormonal imbalances. It's no secret that poultry, cattle, lamb, etc., are pumped with hormones to boost growth, lead to weight gain and enhance overall yield. These hormones are known to interfere with human hormones, too. I remember reading how rBGH, prolactin and progesterone are part of cattle feed. Similarly, chickens are fed oestrogen, progesterone and testosterone for repeated better yields. After all, the fatter the chicken, more are the number of eggs, and more are the profits, right?[61]

Stick to Sattvic Foods

Sattvic food, more popularly known as organic food—if you know the source of the food and how it is prepared when you are consuming it, I think that is sattvic food. Let's take the example of paneer (cottage cheese), which you can buy from a shop or make at home. I would trust the one made at home because I know from where the milk has come, and I can see how it is made in front of my eyes. It basically reduces the possibilities of contamination. Similarly, when you eat at a restaurant, you can't see how it is cooked—is the kitchen hygienic? What taste enhancers are being used? When you eat home-cooked food, you know exactly what you are eating.

Be mindful of what you eat!

Can IVF Clinics Play Foul During Donor Egg IVF?

The answer to this question is both a 'yes' and a 'no'. Let me explain the situations where IVF clinics can misguide a patient.

---

61 K.V. Senthil, C. Rajan, P. Divya and S. Sasikumar, 'Adverse Effects on Consumer's Health Caused by Hormones Administered in Cattle', *International Food Research Journal* 25, no. 1 (2018), pp. 1–10, available at http://www.ifrj.upm.edu.my/25%20(01)%202018/(1).pdf.

Are Clinics Pushing You Towards Egg Donor IVF Cycle?

Understand that the average cost of IVF with an egg donor is higher than the normal route. Also, the chances of success are higher. So, it's a win-win situation for the IVF clinic.

More money + One more success story

You have to *take a sensible call.* Sometimes, this may be the only path for you. I have seen many couples take very long to accept donor egg IVF, and in the process, either waste precious time or continue to harm the body with one failed IVF after another. If your medical background is clearly indicating towards donor cycle, then go for it and save yourself the unnecessary trouble.

Are Clinics Ethical?

A lady from our community once told me that her doctor had emailed her the complete details of the donors, with pictures to choose from. I was stunned. As per government policy, the privacy of both the donor and recipient has to be kept intact. What is the guarantee that clinics of this sort will not leak your details later?

Therefore, speak clearly with your clinic about the privacy clause of the process. Stay away from mushrooming and unethical IVF clinics. Choosing the right IVF clinic is important when opting for egg donor IVF. In fact, as I write this book, the new ART Act, 2022 is being passed and being implemented where the government has made strict mandates for the donor IVF cycles, ensuring that the clinic is following a safe and ethical process. Now, IVF clinics have to take donor egg/sperm from the banks, which will be centralized, much like the blood bank system so that individual clinics/agents can't play foul. This ensures that not only the couple undergoing donor IVF cycle, but also the donor is safeguarded.

Will I Have Twins with IVF?

It is true that IVF pregnancy has more chances of twins because two to three embryos are transferred. However, nothing can be said for sure. I see equal numbers of single and twin baby IVF pregnancies. In fact, you should opt for single embryo transfer as it is less risky than a twin conception, especially if your age is on the higher side and you have associated health risks like BP, diabetes, fibroids, or similar conditions. Twin pregnancies have risks of premature delivery, growth issues of the baby, miscarriage, reduction of one baby at a later stage (when one baby stops growing and threatens the growth of the other one, too). Take an informed decision and don't get swayed by blind optimism.

Can Gender be Determined with IVF?

No, this is not possible. Also, it is illegal to know the gender of your child before your delivery, according to the Pre-Conception and Pre-Natal Diagnostic Techniques (Prohibition of Sex Selection) (PC-PNDT) Act, 2003.

When Can I Get Back to Work? Should I Quit My Job for IVF?

You can get back to work after a week's rest post the embryo transfer. However, you need be in an environment that is not mentally stressful and physically straining. I would recommend not taking the extreme step of quitting your job unless the situation at work is too stressful to handle.

Talk to your boss about your treatment. See if you can work from home.

The idea of quitting your job arises from our social environment, which makes women believe that it is only due to work that they are unable to conceive. And we women beat ourselves up under this pressure.

Also, for me, going to work was a good distraction, and the creative environment kept me positively motivated.

I Am Feeling Dizzy—Am I Already Pregnant?

Implantation happens within seventy-two hours of the embryo transfer so you might begin to feel the early symptoms of pregnancy. On the other hand, dizziness and light-headedness can occur due to heavy medicines and injections. It's best not to jump to conclusions. Wait for the fourteenth day when you do an HCG blood test to confirm the pregnancy. Till then, maintain a healthy diet, sleep well, stay hydrated and well-rested.

Can I Have Sex During the IVF Process?

Yes, you can have sex during the IVF process. However, unlike in IUI process here sex will not lead to increased chances of conception as the mature eggs are already out of your uterus and in the embryology lab for embryo formation process. So, enjoy sex for companionship.

Are Kids Born Out of IVF Normal?

Yes, they are absolutely normal and healthy. The only difference lies in the process of conception, post which the baby grows just like in a normal pregnancy. All the symptoms you experience will be similar to those experienced in a natural pregnancy.

India's first test tube baby, Kanupriya Agarwal, lovingly nicknamed Durga, is now in her forties, and is not only healthy but also the proud mom of a daughter who was conceived normally.[62]

---

[62] M. Somasekhar, 'Kanupriya, India's 1st Test Tube Baby is 43; Mukhopadhyay, Doctor who Helped Her Come to this Life Remains Unsung', *The Siasat Daily*, 3 October 2021, available at https://www.siasat.com/kanupriya-indias-1st-test-tube-baby-is-43-mukhopadhyay-doctor-who-helped-her-come-to-this-life-remains-unsung-2201658/.

Chances of genetic disorders are similar to what you might have in a normal pregnancy. Can we completely control babies born out of normal conception? Don't we have kids with genetic issues and learning disabilities born via natural pregnancy?

What Happens to the Unused Embryos?

Unless you choose to freeze them, unused embryos are discarded as per policy and protocol by the clinics. They will take written consent from you before taking any action.

To conclude, it takes a mind of steel to navigate the labyrinthine process of IVF. You are truly brave. So, pat yourself on the back now that your IVF is done; it is time to sit back and relax for the next two weeks. Pamper yourself and spend some quality couple time together.

'It always seems impossible until it's done.'
— Nelson Mandela

8
How to Prepare for IVF

IVF is all about YOU and your body and mind preparation. Everything else is external and will work in your favour only if the internal works in tandem.

CHECKLIST:

- ☑ Doctor and clinic decided.
- ☑ Initial payment for IVF done.
- ☑ Tentative month of IVF decided.
- ☑ Preparatory diagnostic tests to note baseline parameters done.
- ☑ You both are put on preparatory medicines.

If this is your current checklist, remember not to make this mistake:

- ☒ Don't jump into IVF without preparation

Alternative Methodologies

When my first IVF failed, after a bout of initial depression and exasperation, I started to introspect on what actually went wrong because the doctors had said that everything inside me was okay, physiologically. The embryos were Grade 1, my endometrium lining was also well-formed, and I had taken all medicines and injections as instructed. So, what went wrong?

This question haunted me like madness. It was the missing piece in my IVF puzzle. If I knew what was missing, I could complete the jigsaw. I spent many sleepless nights and anxious days reflecting on this missing piece.

To add to my stress, when I went to the doctor for post-IVF-failure counselling, I was told that doctors generally can't put a finger on what goes wrong, so they will do what they do with all unexplained infertility cases in India—tuberculosis treatment. What? I was bewildered. Isn't tuberculosis a disease prevalent among the lower economic class with issues of malnutrition? In India, tuberculosis is not just a disease, but it is yet another social parameter to judge your lifestyle. Sadly.[63]

My doctor patiently explained that in most cases of unexplained infertility and unexplained IVF failure, a dormant tuberculosis infection is usually an underlying condition, which may show no symptoms until it is time for pregnancy. This infection works against the body and

---

63 G.A. Grace, D.B. Devaleenal and M. Natarajan, 'Genital Tuberculosis in Females', *Indian Journal of Medical Research* 145, no. 4 (2017), pp. 425–36.

negatively impacts one's egg quality or embryo formation or implantation or fallopian tubes or any of the reproductive processes. The doctor also acknowledged that many times, tuberculosis treatment in infertility cure is like throwing darts in the dark. There are many women who have conceived while undergoing TB treatment; however, there is no conclusive study on it.

So, I was put on tuberculosis treatment for six months with a warning that it might have side effects and cause severe gastric issues. In any case, all the IVF hormone injections had completely messed up my stomach. I had already been suffering from intense acidity. Unwillingly, I began with tuberculosis treatment, which is three to four medicines first thing in the morning. I felt extreme nausea, and then throughout the day, I found myself unable to get out of bed. I had no energy, and I would cry incessantly while gulping down the medicines for it was extremely depressing to start the day with medicine like a total 'bimar' (sick person).

This routine continued for a week. I would take the medicines, cry myself to sleep, repeat. Soon, I couldn't take it anymore. I didn't want to bring a child in this depressing environment. Child or no child, this had to stop. My body and mind had given up. I just wanted to run away and hide.

One day, I was mindlessly googling when I came across Auroville. The name and description of the place piqued my interest. Nestled in Puducherry, Auroville is an international township based on the philosophy of Mother and Sri Aurobindo. A universal, experimental township progressing towards creating an ideal and sustainable society that lives in peace and harmony.

They had an option to apply as volunteer. It was close to Chennai, where I was residing at that time, and thus, seemed like the perfect escape from my current situation. I was approached by Danny from Wellpaper, a non-governmental organization (NGO) working with Tsunami-hit women, training them to make products from old newspaper and making a sustainable living out of it. Danny offered me free lunch and free housesitting offer in exchange for volunteering to help him with his website content and digital marketing. I couldn't have asked for a better deal. I was ready to experience something. I was anxious, but it was a good kind of anxiety after a long time.

On my first night in Auroville, I was scared. I had never stayed alone; plus, my family was apprehensive of this trip, even to the extent that they thought I am done with my marriage and was planning to divorce my husband, and was thus using this trip as a cover-up. The truth was that my partner and I had hit rock bottom in our relationship. This infertility treatment had taken a toll on our marriage. Incidentally, on my first night in Auroville, I got my hands on a small booklet called *Fear* written by Sri Aurbindo and the Mother.

Here are some lines from the book:

> Fear plays a preeminent role in the human experience and manifests itself in diverse forms in our lives. Excessive indulgence in fear is counter-productive because that propagates vibrations which may attract the very phenomena that we cringe from, according to the Mother.

How to Prepare for IVF

Question: Why does one feel afraid?

Mother: I suppose it is because one is egoistic.
There are three reasons. First, an excessive concern about one's security. Next, what one does not know always gives an uneasy feeling which is translated in the consciousness by fear. And above all, one doesn't have the habit of a spontaneous trust in the Divine. If you look into things sufficiently deeply, this is the true reason. There are people who do not even know that That exists, but one could tell them in other words, 'You have no faith in your destiny' or 'You know nothing about Grace'—anything whatever, you may put it as you like, but the root of the matter is a lack of trust. If one always had the feeling that it is the best that happens in all circumstances, one would not be afraid.[64]

Fear, yes.

I had found the missing piece of my IVF puzzle. It was the fear of treading this unknown path, my fear of what society would think of me if I was childless, fear of me being alone in life without having someone to shower my selfless love on, my fear of the future and the present, and past fears. I had a realization—I was engulfed in many fears at multiple levels of my being.

---

64 Sri Aurobindo & The (d.i. Mira Alfassa) Mother, Fear and Its Overcoming, (Pondicherry: Verlag und Fachbuchhandel Wilfried Schuh Auro Media, 2018).

There was no turning back from there. I decided to have an open mind and heart to experience new things without fear. I started to work on my fears. I slowly began to train my mind to stay in the present.

I met Mallika in Auroville. Born in France, she had travelled to India in the eighties because she had been inspired by Mother's teachings. Since then, she has been in Auroville, practising healing therapies. She worked with me closely to bring back my balance. She is my fairy godmother. I experienced acupuncture and moksha (Chinese therapy) under her supervision and started preparing for my next round of IVF.

I tried everything, from past life regression, crystal healing for chakra balancing, to group Om chanting, acupuncture, flower cure therapy, moksha, aura balancing, and full moon meditation.

The time I spent in Auroville helped me restore my balance and gave me an opportunity to work on my subconscious, connect with my unadulterated personal being, bring a clarity to where I am and what actually makes me happy, and reinforce my trust in the universe. This experience came at a critical juncture in my fertility journey and helped in many ways for my next attempt at IVF.

Alternative methodologies can be effectively used as holistic, complementary, and alternative approaches to pre-conception IVF preparation. IVF is a complex treatment process that tests the body, mind and relationships, and you need to be properly armed to tackle its many aspects, especially IVF failure. About 60 to 70 per cent IVFs fail, and on an average, a couple needs about two-and-a-half cycles of IVF to be successful. Preparation for IVF is thus crucial.

Choose alternative methodologies that suit you or a combination of a few based on your philosophy, comfort, lifestyle and personality. The idea is to prepare yourself—your body—so that it can handle the pressure, and also the mind which quietly faces the brunt of it all.

Alternative methodologies work when practised as complementary and holistic to IVF treatment and have shown remarkable results, thereby improving chances of success.[65]

On being asked if he suggests alternative methodologies to his patients, Dr Munjaal, an IVF doctor from Mumbai, said:

> There are no scientific or conclusive theories correlating IVF and alternative treatment, so as an allopathy doctor I don't suggest them. However, I don't ever discourage them either. Anything that gives my patients peace, calm and sanity during this time is good. As long as it doesn't cause harm there is nothing to worry. Most of my patients are quite happy with acupuncture and acupressure therapies.[66]

---

65   Y. Zhang, Y. Fu, F. Han, H. Kuang, M. Hu and X. Wu, 'The Effect of Alternative Medicine on Subfertile Women with In Vitro Fetilization', *Evidence-Based Complementary and Alternative Medicine* 2014, no. 2014 (2014), available at https://www.ncbi.nlm.nih.gov/pmc/articles/PMC3914344/.

66   Interview with Dr Munjaal, IVF doctor from Mumbai.

Ayurveda

The Ayurveda approach complements the IVF treatment phase quite successfully. Ayurveda takes care of all aspects of a human being. It is a holistic way of life. Ayurveda preconception care prepares a couple both physically and mentally. This holistic approach ensures better success chances. Again, due to lack of substantive research, there are no conclusive numbers to prove this theory, but based on simple logic and real-life experiences, the combination of Ayurveda and IVF is complementary.

Our hectic lifestyles are rather stressful, which is a major cause for infertility. Along with lifestyle habits such as alcohol consumption and environmental toxicity affecting sperm count, and sperm's quality and motility, it also depletes the zinc level in the body, whereas in females, it affects ovulation and menstruation, leading to the hypothalamic pituitary ovarian dysfunction.[67]

In Ayurveda, Panchakarma (a method to cleanse the body of all unwanted toxins using five deep cleansing procedures) therapy acts at the hormonal level, keeping hormones at normal levels. Thus, hormonal defects in infertility can be rectified by Panchakarma procedures. This therapy also helps in the removal of accumulated toxins.

---

67 R.P. Sindhu and S. Sivaramakrishnapillai, 'Preconception Care in Ayurveda', Journal of Indian system of Medicine 7, no. 2 (2019), pp. 90–92, available at https://www.joinsysmed.com/article.asp?issn=2320-4419;year=2019;volume=7;issue=2;spage=90;epage=92;aulast=Sindhu;type=0.

For PCOS[68] or male infertility,[69] Ayurveda is highly recommended. However, in cases where there is a structural anomaly like inverted ovaries or azoospermia (nil sperms), Ayurveda can't do much.

Ayurveda can help with building the endometrium lining and preparing the uterus to accept the embryo, which is a critical step in the success of IVF. In the male partner, the improvement of sperm count, quality and motility will ensure quality embryo creation. Most importantly, Ayurveda therapies help reduce stress and anxiety that can't be ignored during an IVF process but need to be in control for the proper facilitation of IVF.

Usually, doctors will ask you to lose weight to aid in conception. Here, Ayurveda can immensely assist. Treatments like Shodananga and Snehapana help control weight issues. When body weight reduces, menstrual cycle gets normalized, and ovulation is regulated. Dr Rani, an Ayurveda infertility specialist practising in Delhi says, 'When a woman who has infertility issues comes to us, we don't immediately zone into the pelvic area. According to Ayurvedic principles, we have to analyse her complete health status.'[70]

---

68 D. Mishra and M. Sinha, 'Ayurvedic Management of Polycystic Ovarian Syndrome (Infertility Queen)', *Journal of Research and Education in Indian Medicine* 14, no. 1 (2008), pp. 33–40, available at https://www.jreim-ayushjournal.com/fulltext/82-1433809662.pdf.

69 N. Vyas, K. Gamit and M. Raval, 'Male Infertility: A Major Problem Worldwide and its Management in Ayurveda', *Pharma Science Monitor* 9, no. 1 (2018), pp. 446–69.

70 Interview with Dr Rani, Ayurveda Infertility Specialist, New Delhi.

The Seven Dhatus

According to Ayurveda, there are seven dhatus or tissues in our body, according to Ayurveda. They are: rasa (plasma), rakta (blood), mamsa (flesh), medas (muscle), asthi (fat), majja (bone) and shukra (marrow/nerve and reproductive tissue). Shukra is the last and final one, and the most refined because it is responsible for reproductive health. Interestingly, all the seven dhatus work in a sequential way, starting from rasa dhatu. Thus, we can't pick or correct any one tissue in isolation. So, to get to fixing issues with the shukra dhatu (which when off balance causes infertility issues), we need to fix the whole chain and make everything work cohesively.

Rasa dhatu is made out of good food and good digestion. So, you need to start from the very beginning, trying to balance the doshas, and then, gradually reach the most complex shukra dhatu. In Ayurveda, a diagnosis of imbalance is figured out based on three body types (or doshas) namely kapha, vata and pitta. Treatment begins by working on metabolism (rasa dhatu), and sequentially moves ahead to improve tissue formation, detoxing and tonification (rebuilding) of the internal organs; all of this will eventually show results in fertility enhancement. This process usually takes three months. So, a couple should plan to start Ayurveda treatments at least three months before IVF to optimize the benefits.

As a general methodology in Ayurveda for balancing fertility health, first detoxification (cleaning) is done, followed by tonification.

To detoxify your system, based on your dosha type (kapha, vata or pitta), panchakarma treatment is advised. For example, if kapha is dominant or imbalanced, vamana (medical vomiting where a medicated drink is given and you vomit under guidance to clean the body thoroughly) is done, if pitta imbalance is seen, virechana (therapeutic purgation) is the suitable panchakarma methodology, if vata is aggravated, basti (enema) is advised. You can also be a combination of doshas. For example, I am more kapha but at the same time display vata qualities. Out of the five methodologies of panchakarma—vamana, virechana, basti, nasya, and rakta moksha—suitable ones are chosen based on your dosha and of the dominant dosha type.

After a few sessions of detoxification, the tonifying or rebuilding phase wherein specific gynaecological procedures are executed begins. Uttar basti is an extremely effective treatment specific to gynaecological problems like urinary tract infections (UTIs), tubal blockage, PCOS, abortions, unexplained infertility, endometriosis and menstrual inconsistencies. 'In fact, uttar basti has amazing results with opening blocked fallopian tubes', says Dr Swathi Ashutosh certified Bachelor of Ayurvedic Medicine and Surgery (BAMS) doctor with MS in Ayurveda, and practising as a consultant with Fertility Dost.[71]

In this process, medicated oils are lightly massaged on the stomach (snehan), then steam is given (swedan), followed by uttar basti, wherein medicated oils are administered

---

71 Interview with Dr Swathi Ashutosh, BAMS Doctor, MS in Ayurveda, Consultant with Fertility Dost.

through a rubber catheter into the cervix. Usually, three cycles of uttar basti with three to four sessions per cycle will show visible results. This treatment helps women with thin endometrium lining issues, thereby enhancing implantation success rate.

Ayurveda procedures of panchakarma and oral medicines help regulate the menstrual cycle. They also correct LH and FSH levels.

Ayurvedic Treatment for Male Infertility

The branch of Ayurveda dealing with the sexual wellbeing of men is called Vajikarana. Male infertility issues like sperm count, motility and form issues can be corrected through panchakarma treatment. Similar rules and processes will be applied, wherein based on your dosha, a particular treatment will be advised. For example, a sperm count issues usually points to vata imbalance; if motility is weak, it means that kapha dosha is predominant, and for form related issues, it is vata-pitta disorder.

Regular exercise, yoga, and eating balanced meals helps keep the mind, body and soul balanced. Include the following yoga asanas in your daily yoga practice.

1. padmasana (lotus pose),
2. paschimottanasana (seated forward bend),
3. bhujangasana (cobra pose),
4. sarvangasana (shoulder stand),
5. praivritta trikonasana (twisted triangle pose).

Figure 8.1: Yoga to Improve Male Fertility

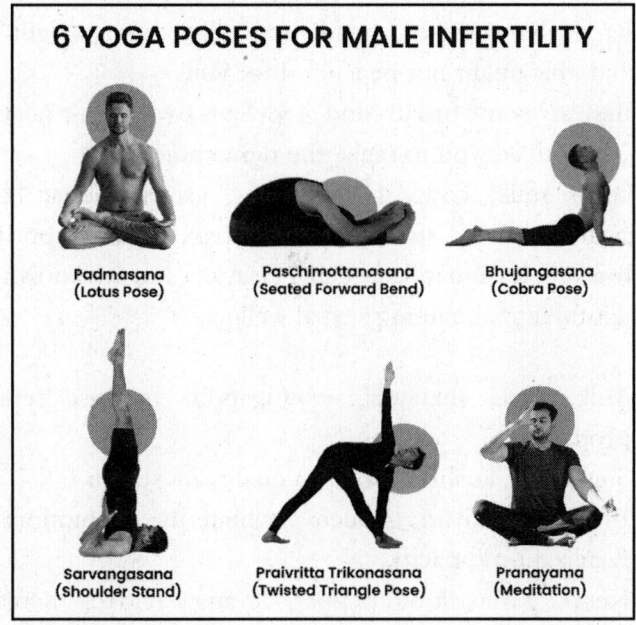

Source: Designed by the author, using images from www.shutterstock.com.

Ayurvedic Medicines and Food

Ayurveda is a very specific science catering to your individual needs, combining multiple factors like your doshas, your current physical and emotional state, etc. What may be highly effective for you might not work for someone else. As per Ayurvedic shastra, an individual treatment approach is stressed upon. So, it is best to consult an Ayurvedic doctor and get a customized plan, especially when dealing with infertility.

For example, the herb shatvari can help increase fertility but has a tendency to lead to weight gain. Now if you have kapha dosha and are already struggling with weight or thyroid, this might not be a good for you.

Here are some broad food guidelines to set a perspective and to motivate you to make the right choice.

Cow's milk, cow's ghee, honey, ashwagandha, bala, shatavari, triphala, shilajitu, musali pak, chyawanaprasha, vrishya vati, kushmanda avaleha, rasayana vati are known to be helpful in maintaining sexual wellness.

1. Milk, ghee, shatavari, ashwagandha increase semen production.
2. Sugarcane, kushtha work on quality of semen.
3. Brahmi, shatavari, guduchi facilitate the promotion of fertilization capacity.
4. Kesar, garlic, long pepper, lavanga (clove) increase libido.
5. Nutmeg, ashwagandha, chandana prevent premature ejaculation.
6. Dry fruits like almonds, walnuts, black currants, figs, dates, etc. with milk serve as vajikarana.
7. Black gram included in the pre-conception diet is a rich source of folic acid, proteins and fibers.
8. Rice contains more of carbohydrates and rice bran contains vitamin B complex, which is easily digestible.
9. Milk provides calcium.
10. Ghee has properties of imparting strength, improving tonicity, and nourishing the body.

How to Prepare for IVF

11. The consumption of masha, tila taila, milk, and ghee by couples will help in the production of efficient sperm and ovum, which will result in good progeny.
12. For better endometrium/uterine lining, a good diet that increases blood level in body like spinach (palak), pomegranate (anar) and coconut water is required.

Do You Know How Critical the Endometrium Lining Is?

Figure 8.2: The Cycle of Blood

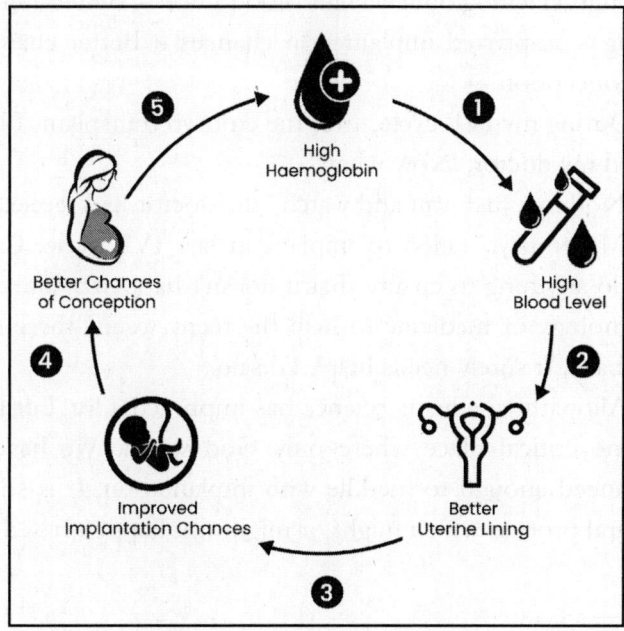

Source: Created by the author.

'Problems with the endometrium lining contributes to 30 per cent of IVF failures', says Dr Sonia Malik , senior IVF consultant from, New Delhi.[72]

For an embryo to successfully implant, the uterine lining is critical. The ideal thickness should be between 10 and 15 mm. Medication is usually provided during the IVF cycle to thicken this lining.

The uterine lining is formed by the blood flowing into the uterus. Thus, your haemoglobin levels are crucial. Many women are asked to increase their haemoglobin levels during the initial treatment stages. Do you now see the whole cycle?

High Haemoglobin – High Blood Level – Better uterine lining – Improved implantation chances – Better chances of conception

During my IVF cycle, after the embryo transplant, I had asked my doctor, 'Now what?'

'Nothing. Just wait and watch,' the doctor had replied.

'My embryo failed to implant in last IVF cycle. Can't we do anything to ensure that it doesn't happen again? No technology or medicine to help the teeny-weeny three-day old baby. It surely needs help', I'd said.

'Allopathy medicine science has improved a lot, but this is one critical place where only God works. We haven't advanced enough to meddle with implantation. It is still a natural process which might or might not happen based on

---

[72] Interview with Dr Sonia Malik, senior IVF Consultant, New Delhi.

How to Prepare for IVF

a lot of factors, none of which we can accurately pinpoint or manage,' the doctor had replied.

So, now you know how critical endometrium lining is.

Choosing the Right Ayurveda Specialist

A word of caution here: choose an Ayurveda clinic or doctor with experience in handling infertility patients because the treatment procedures are specific to the problem. Today, there are Ayurveda centres at every nukkad, all selling panchakarma treatments like another day in spa. You need to be careful. Common ayurvedic treatments like Abhyangam or Shirodhara might not be particularly effective for fertility enhancement.

Box 8.1: Quick Ayurveda Checklist

> ☑ Ayurvedic treatment need a minimum of three months to show results.
> ☑ Go to an Ayurvedic doctor with experience in handling infertility and gynaecology cases.
> ☑ Ayurveda is not a generalized science. It is a personalized treatment and will vary as per your body type. So don't trust generic, off-the-shelf advice.
> ☑ Basic rules of good food, nutrition and exercise apply to all.

Source: Created by the author.

Naturopathy and Yoga

Naturopathy and yoga are nature-aligned lifestyle programmes that correct imbalances and reset the body and mind back to its natural settings. It is like setting the factory reset button on your mobile.

Naturopathy focuses on enhancing your body and mind's balance, restoring it back to its natural state, optimizing their functionality quite similar to how we reset our phones to factory setting and it is as good as new. It is basically an experiential process with the ultimate goal of lifestyle modifications to cure the physical ailments from the root itself.

Naturopathy can help with any lifestyle-related/modification issue such as obesity, PCOS, sleep imbalances, sperm quality and other neuro-functional modifications, hypothyroidism and other hormonal imbalances, etc. It also works in cases where structural correction though surgeries, etc. is required.

Naturopathy uses a three-phase approach:

(1) Elimination of toxins/wastes from the body.
(2) Rebalancing the functional elements.
(3) Nourishment as required to enhance the functions.

Dr Jayachandra Thampi, a Naturopath practitioner, said in an interview that these can be achieved through various techniques like:

1. Nutrition/dietetics: Calorie-restricted/time-restricted nutrition, high plant-based dietary approach, educating

yourself on food quantity and quality in the daily life as per the need, specific supplementation (food).
2. Water/Hydro therapies: Local and general baths using water at various temperatures to enhance organ functions (for example: a hip bath is a bath given locally to the pelvic area in a tub combined with specific exercises to enhance pelvic floor functions and thus, address local/specific area needs).
3. Physical therapies: Massages and other manipulative therapies to improve circulation, muscle and structural tonicity, etc.
4. Yoga: Ensures overall physical and mental wellbeing is an unavoidable part of the programme.
5. Acupuncture: This is especially in certain conditions like sleep, hormonal and immune-related functions, stress, etc.

Since it is a lifestyle intervention programme, couples should start naturopathy, combined with yoga sessions, a minimum of three months before an IVF procedure, thus giving the body ample time for preparation. Also, I would emphasize that both partners participate together, primarily because it gives men the opportunity to understand what women go through and it also creates a bond of togetherness through the process.

IVF is an invasive, complex and draining process, so careful prior preparation is imperative. Naturopathy can be an essential element of the pre-IVF preparation. Since it is a non-pharmacological intervention and management programme, it can easily be implemented with IVF. In fact, it could help minimize some of the adverse side effects, undesirable body inflammations, and mind fluctuations when you undergo IVF due to various hormonal and other interventions.

Look for a naturopathy centre or a doctor with considerable years of experience. Jindal Nature Cure in Bangalore, Arya Vaidya Sala in Kottakal and Parmarth Nature Cure in Rishikesh are some of the notable centres in India.

Box 8.2: Quick Tips

1. Maintain ideal weight and height.
2. Wake up before sunrise.
3. Specific pelvic floor exercises with breathing (yoga and other regular exercises).
4. Ensure whole spine flexibility is maintained as many a time upper back rigidity leads to improper metabolism, especially fat.
5. In short, sweating daily is a must (moderate intensity exercise only).
6. Hip baths/sitz baths (normal temperature bath given locally to pelvic area for ten to fifteen minutes, followed by pelvic exercises) help enhance pelvic floor and reproductive organ functions very much.
7. Minimize sugar in all forms in the diet (whole cereal organic products are fine).
8. Reduce salt in the diet.
9. Once a week **NO GRAIN DIET**.
10. Lots of water (3+ litres a day).

How to Prepare for IVF

11. Non-sugary snacks (if snacking is needed).
12. Keep an eight-hour food timing (eat food within eight hours from the first meal to the last meal of the day).
13. Ideally, wake up before sunrise; and the first main meal (breakfast) must be after one hour minimum.
14. Once-a-week/fortnight fasting on fruits and dried fruits are beneficial (**NO CEREAL DIET**).
15. Sunbathing with mild joint movements helps boost Vitamin D levels, and thus, many internal functions, including hormonal and metabolic functions. Follow with a citrus fruit juice like lime/lemon.
16. Deep sleep must be ensured between 11 p.m. and 4 a.m. (to get this, go to bed by 10 p.m. latest and wake up after 5 a.m. only).
17. Breathing exercises help to counter stress and metabolic dullness. Fast breathing exercises are useful (learn from teachers and only then practise).
18. Minimize the use of medicines like pain killers and other over-the-counter medicines for inflammations, cold, etc.
19. Castor oil packs on the lower abdomen (apply castor oil and wrap with a cotton cloth followed by water bag compress) are helpful.
20. Once-a-week massages or any such muscle stress-managing activity.

Source: Created by the author.

Box 8.3: Some Additional Tips for Men

- In addition, smoking must be stopped; alcohol must be stopped at least on trial months.
- Dried fruits, seeds like pumpkin and sunflower must be added in the diet. Soybeans may be minimized.
- Moderate to high intensity exercise is must.

Source: Created by the author.

Acupuncture

I was introduced to acupuncture by Mallika a sixty-year-old lady, originally from France, who came to India in her late twenties and then settled in Auroville (Puducherry) to follow her spiritual pursuits.

The therapy room was small with a single bed covered in a clean white sheet and white flowers decorated around it, two chairs, a small table in the corner, with an aromatic incense stick burning, and light-yellow coloured curtain dancing with the breeze. There was something good about the energy of the place. The moment I entered the room, I already felt relaxed. A petite lady wearing a white salwar suit with an amazing glow on her face entered the room and made me sit in this comfortable chair. She asked me a few questions and in no time, tears started rolling down my eyes as I shared my story with her. Later, she performed the acupuncture therapy, and I don't know about anything else, but I surely felt light and had something in me which said, You will sail through this!'

Traditional Chinese Medicine (TCM) is about 3,000 years old, starting from the Zhou Dynasty of China.

TCM is the art of preventing and/or treating a disease by using different techniques. It is based on the Chinese postulate that there is an energy flow (qi) in every living being that is responsible for life. This energy flow is mainly influenced by the action of the sun (Yang) and the moon (Yin). While modern science is based on symptoms and its cure, TCM is a holistic study of medicine.

Acupuncture is a branch of TCM. Using a technique of needles which are inserted in selected points on the body or along certain channels called meridians, it helps to keep or regain the balance of qi. For example, acupuncture can be used to isolate a blockage, clear it, stimulate reproductive functions, disperse the energy.

Acupuncture works in two ways—through the traditional and the modern approach. An acupuncturist can use an individual approach or combine the two. In case of infertility management, the best approach is to integrate the modern system. The treatment of acupuncture works when the circulation of qi and blood has been restored, modified, or put in balance, according to Chinese laws like Yin and Yang and pulse reading.

Male Infertility and Acupuncture

Male potency is important for the success of any fertility treatment, especially IVF. Some of the issues that can be managed with acupuncture are:

- Flaccidity of the penis or incomplete erection,
- Spasms,
- Pruritis of testicles,
- Urethritis,
- Sexual excess,
- Insufficiency or seminal discharge,
- Contracted testicles,
- Coldness of the testicular sack,
- Diabetes,
- Dysfunction of the Autonomic Nervous System.

For Female Infertility

For women, impotency mostly refers to a psychological or energy block that stops them from achieving orgasm during sexual intercourse. Classic symptoms are feelings of extreme and constant cold, lack of desire for sexual act, and frequent issues with genital parts (like urinary tract issues, swelling or itching of the vagina, white discharge, foul smell).

Acupuncture works directly with the energy levels of the body (needles are inserted at the exact meridians) with the aim of harmonizing the energy (known as Yin and Yang). The best thing about acupuncture is that it works on both the body and the mind. You will feel lighter (reduced stress) and high on energy (increased blood circulation to the reproductive organs).

Right Time to Get Acupuncture Sessions

'A good acupuncturist is the one who cures those who are not yet sick.'

If you decide to start acupuncture treatment, do so as soon as you decide to plan conception. Before you plan on getting pregnant, both you and your partner can check your general health and the health of your sexual organs with a few sessions. It also means that you would not want to wait for problems of infertility to emerge later.

But if you already suffer from infertility, contact specialists in this field along with conducting of medical tests immediately. In cases of infertility, acupuncture is best when started at an early stage for it helps avoid stress, anxiety, depression to set in.

The right time to conduct acupuncture sessions is just before an IVF cycle. It is not advisable to go for acupuncture treatment after embryo transfer till the end of the first trimester, if you conceive.

Make sure to find the right acupuncturist. A needle in the wrong place is even known to cause irreversible damage. Only if you trust the acupuncturist fully, you should go ahead with them.

Astrology

I was going to start my IVF when Soumen, who believes in astrology cajoled me to pay a visit to this family astrologer. It seemed like he was looking for some reassurance. The astrologer looked at our charts and said that though he can see a baby in our near future, there are also some hurdles. Well! The way to negotiate the hurdles was to wear an expensive stone ring. Soumen fell for it totally. Just two days before the IVF, instead of focusing on us, he was busy arranging for the money to buy the stone. I did wear the ring and still my IVF failed.

I don't want to be hypocritical or preachy. I have been there, done that! Now, I don't get bullied into buying an expensive stone; a good astrologer would never do that to you. If going to an astrologer gives you some kind of solace and reassurance, do it, but don't get blinded by faith. It is like walking on thin ice. Trust me, if it is about reaching out to God, a simple honest prayer will also do the task.

Box 8.4: Points to Remember about Astrologers

> ☑ Don't get used by them.
> ☑ Don't fall into a trap.
> ☑ Go for the reliable ones only.
> ☑ Use your logic and gut feeling.
> ☑ Don't pin all your hopes on their predictions.
> ☑ Go with an open mind and don't be bogged down by desperation.
> ☑ It should not distress you any further. If it relaxes at some level then go for it.

Source: Created by the author.
Disclaimer: To go or not to go is your personal choice.

Learn to Control Your Mind

Our mind is the real culprit here that needs to be controlled for the IVF treatment to go through successfully. Once we decide to undergo IVF, our expectation becomes sky high. We think that it is some magic pill that will miraculously reset everything around us.

1. Trust the process, don't fear it.
2. Have realistic expectations.
3. Focus on preparing well for the complete process and not just on the outcome (over-hoping for positive pregnancy).
4. Teach your mind to be resilient and patient.

Manage Stress and Anxiety

Stress is not a bad condition. Everyone gets a basic level of stress, which is fine, and doesn't hamper the routine of life; but the problem begins when we don't know how to put a stop to that stress and keep stretching it like blood pressure (which is essential for life, but high pressure is bad). We cannot avoid stress (external situations), but we can equip ourselves with better stress management systems.

We cannot control the medical reasons for IVF failure, but we can definitely learn how to manage stress.

The best coping mechanism I found was following the sun. A set routine always helps to calm the mind down. Even if you don't feel like it, owing to the mind being in a mess, force the body to follow the routine with discipline, and you will see that slowly the mind will learn to follow. Wake up just before sunrise, then do some warm-up exercises (walk or yoga), then eat a good breakfast, lunch should be a full meal (according to Naturopathy, during noon the sun is at the peak, and thus, the body needs more energy, and a heavy lunch is ideal), and end the day with a light dinner in the evening to let the body calm down. After sunset, allow your body and mind to slowly wind down and sleep.

Take each day as it comes. Plan well, but don't overthink, overtly focusing on the outcome. The infertility journey will make your feel that you are losing control. In such a situation, instead of panicking, keep daily doable goals for yourself. Achieve those goals to get some sense of control back and be happy about achieving those smaller goals. Most of the days, out of anxiety, I used to be on the couch mindlessly watching TV for hours together. The only excuse I had was that I am not feeling well. It was a loop in which I had got stuck. I wasn't feeling well, so I just let it be without doing anything, and I continued to keep feeling unwell; and most of this feeling unwell was mental, not physical. Then one fine day, I decided to give myself a goal of going on an evening walk for at least thirty minutes. I pushed myself to change, wear my shoes, literally thrusting myself out of the door. I felt good.

A change of location always helps to distract the mind and take the stress off. It gives you time to break the pattern of stress and rethink. Especially if you live in the madness of a metro city, a trip to a nice location will do you good.

Stress invariably impacts our metabolism. Ensure that you are eating right and adding probiotics and fibre to your diet to keep your bowel movements regular.

There is a life outside trying for pregnancy. Focus on that. Don't put all your energy into your fertility journey. Remember, it is just a part of life and not life itself. This distinction will help you channelize your energies better.

Try Meditation

I found meditation techniques handy during the process of my embryo transfer. There is a lot going on during this process—you are in an OT surrounded by doctors and nurses in scrubs, you are not under anaesthesia, the ultrasound machine is set over you, the doctor is getting the vial ready, your bladder is full, and you are anxious like hell. But you must stay calm because it is a process of extreme precision, and the calmer you are, better the doctor can perform. The embryo must reach as close to the uterus as possible. Staying calm amid everything is critical.

And meditation will help you immensely at this stage.

I won't say control your stress and anxiety during the IVF process for that is not practical advice. What you can do is *manage stress and anxiety to keep them within limits*. Meditation or relaxing techniques help greatly in managing anxiety. It is best to practise guided meditation under an expert.

Another reason why you should try meditation is the theory of beej sanskar (an Ayurvedic theory on reproductive health and conception), which says that the thoughts that you have during conception sets the baby's unconscious. Essentially, this means that the parent's psychological state during fertilization has an impact on the foetus.

'If the couple is happy during intercourse the child born out of it would be Sattvika, if frustrated then Rajasika and if sorrowful then Tamasika', says Dr V.N.K. Usha, Preconceptional Care in Ayurveda.[73]

Thus, there is definitely a correlation between implantation, your emotional wellness and the first seeds of unconscious psychological wellness of the foetus. Now, look at the brighter side. During normal conception, you don't know what mood you are in when fertilization happens. However, in IVF, you know each step of the way. All you need to do is have a good emotional and psychological quotient during the process and manifest your dream child.

In hindsight, I feel that my first IVF failed because I was too anxious and totally messed up in my mind. Clearly, at that time, I was so frustrated with the journey that I forgot to enjoy the process of baby-making; I forgot why I really wanted to have a child. It seemed that I was in a rush to prove to society that I was not 'infertile', and that can never be the right reason, right?

During my second IVF, I had learnt to be resilient. I was armed with tips to manage anxiety, and most importantly, I wanted to have a baby for the right reasons. I was calmer. Though it is too soon to brag about my loved one who is

---

[73] Dr .K. Usha, Preconception Care in Ayurveda (New Delhi: Chaukhamba Sanskrit Pratishthan, 2007).

Work on Past Guilt

Why me? What wrong did I do?

These are the most frequent and haunting questions that mostly women try to answer, mostly in vain, during their fertility treatment journey.

Shikha, a twenty-five-year-old software engineer from Ajmer had an unplanned pregnancy, and she got an abortion because it was too early in the marriage. Years later, when she was ready to enter motherhood, she met the biggest roadblock, infertility. She kept beating herself up. 'I had aborted my natural pregnancy that's why God is punishing me today. I am a bad person. I don't deserve to be a mom. I committed a sin.'[74]

When I had my first miscarriage, a close relative who came to check on my wellbeing, said, 'One miscarriage is fine. Don't worry. You must think about leaving your job. I saw you the other day coming so late from office and thought to myself, this is not good, but didn't want to say anything for the fear of being nosy.'

This thought of my job causing an advanced miscarriage (fourth month) stayed with me as guilt for a long time. I believed it and was punitive to myself for being so reckless.

---

[74] Interview with Shikha, a twenty-five-year-old software engineer, Ajmer.

Guilt kept building in my subconscious and my self-esteem kept falling. I didn't realize then that all this was being caused by a bigger socially prejudiced environment because I was naturally over-sensitive and vulnerable during that time. So, these silly things had an impact on me. Holding the woman responsible for infertility is intrinsic to a stereotypical social belief system, and you get caught in this trap because you have also grown up within it. Thus, blaming yourself becomes common practice.

But you need to stop with the self-blame and guilt to successfully move ahead in the journey of fertility. Can you move ahead if your feet are chained?

You need to consciously weed such thoughts out. You may take the help of a psychologist, life coach or a mentor. This exercise also helps build positive thought and energy, much needed to sail through IVF.

Have a Plan B

It is natural for you to pin all your hopes on IVF. You have waited long, failed a few times, felt desperate, oscillated between hope and anxiety, and borne taunts of society and indescribable pain.

I know it will break your heart to even think that this won't work before it has even started. But the truth is that subconsciously you are constantly experiencing fear and anxiety of failure, even though from the outside you try to show you are normal and strong. When your inner self is not calm, it leads to intermittent bouts of anxiety where you find yourself happy in one moment and then sad for no comprehensible reason in another moment. This will fatigue your mind soon.

It is natural to feel fearful because a lot is at stake.

So, what do you do?

The solution here is to get practical and have a Plan B.

What is Plan B?

Plan B is simply a concrete plan of what you will do if your IVF cycle fails. No emotions attached. Just practical things like:

1. **Book a vacation:** And hey, if you get pregnant, all you need to do is cancel the booking. Won't you do that happily? But if the cycle fails, a vacation will give you a much-required breather, and the change of environment will help restore your balance.
2. **Conscious effort to look for an alternative route**: When I was having my second IVF, I had promised myself that if this one failed, I would not waste time crying and getting depressed. I'd begin the process of adoption the very next day. I am not saying that adoption is an alternative to a failed IVF. However, you need to have an alternate plan, which can be anything that suits your situation—thinking about being child-free or the next treatment path. The core point here is to stay logical, practical and conscious. Avoid falling into an emotional trap. Be a doer.

3. **Get to work**: If you are not already working, take up any work, even freelance, or go work voluntarily with an NGO, or teach in a school. Do something that keeps you busy, motivated, and makes you feel that you are doing something substantial.
4. **Try a hobby:** Join an art class or a dance school. Surprise yourself. Do something completely random and push yourself out of your comfort zone. The adrenalin rush you will experience will help you forget your pain and teach you to live in the present. And the joy of accomplishing something new or having a new experience will give you the happy booster dose you need to stay afloat.

These are some suggestions, but the idea is to have a tentative plan with actionable points to help you, if you need it.

Food and Diet

When I asked Dr Parul Katiyar, Senior Fertility Consultant, New Delhi if she advises alternative treatments to her patients, she emphasized that more than anything else, she advises IVF couples on healthy eating and nutrition to prepare well.

Let's just get this out of the way—there is nothing like one diet that can be called a 'fertility diet'. The basic thumb rules of food and diet remain the same. Yes, there are some foods that you should take and some to completely avoid to manage specific issues like PCOS, sperm quality, endometrium lining, thyroid, period issues, and the like. However, there is no generic 'one diet suits all' type of mantra.

It is good to see a nutritionist and get a customized plan based on your current lifestyle, exact medical issues, and the goal you aim at achieving as a part of your preconception or IVF planning. There are many types of diet consultations available based on different philosophies—Ayurveda-inspired, sattvic foods, ketogenic, gluten-free, vegan, intermittent fasting, etc.

How would you know which one is the right one here?

Remember, the aim is **NOT QUICK WEIGHT LOSS** but to have a healthy diet that keeps your energy levels high, hormones balanced, blood circulation improved, and provides the required nutrients to enhance overall reproductive health.

There is no shortcut to achieving pregnancy. Thus:

- Avoid any fad diet.
- Avoid crash dieting.
- Avoid following anything and everything you read on Google.
- Don't try anything too drastic or new.

One of my community members, Ruhina (name changed), was advised by her doctor to lose weight while being on her fertility journey as her thyroid level was on the higher side. It was a general advice for wellbeing, apart from a whole lot of tests and other protocols. At home, her in-laws were curious about the doctor's advice. 'The doctor has said everything is fine with us. She just needs to lose some weight,' her husband replied.

All hell broke loose. It was naively assumed that weight was the only roadblock between Ruhina and her pregnancy. Ruhina's mother-in-law took it very seriously and limited her food intake. If Ruhina reached out for a second roti, she was met with frowns. She was made to join the most expensive gym in their locality. In her zeal, she went to the gym in the morning and aerobics in the evening. Her life was caught between exercise routines and absolutely no food. As a result of this extreme lifestyle, she had vertigo and complete blackout, and her glucose level fell so low that she had to be admitted to the hospital.

You need to understand that while weight is surely an issue, the bigger goal is to achieve pregnancy for which you need stable hormone levels, a healthy uterus, and a happy heart. You just need to maintain a healthy body mass index (BMI) level.

You need a diet that can focus on **YOU**:

1. Go for personalized diet consultation with a fertility nutritionist.
2. Moderation and balance are key.
3. Pick a diet style that is sustainable over time.
4. Follow the diet together as a couple.
5. Enjoy the diet and don't eat as a punishment. If you don't like anything, have an open conversation with your nutritionist and look for an alternative.
6. Don't give up quickly. Keep trying.

Keep a balance of folic acid, iron, protein and calcium in your diet as a general baseline for your pre-conception diet. Again, personally, I have issues when I increase my iron intake. It just messes with my stomach. However, initially, I was told by some well-meaning person that I needed to take more iron. I was low on haemoglobin, too. So, I upped my iron intake, all the while ignoring side effects like constipation and bloating. But I pushed on because how would I become a mother if I couldn't endure a little bit of discomfort and pain, right?

This is all BULLSHIT.

Don't repeat my mistakes. There is no report card of life and there is nobody standing at the end to cheer you. It is your life, your body, and you know it best. You don't want to be an unhappy mom when you finally get there.

You must carefully observe your diet and note how your body is responding. Don't push yourself unnecessarily. Check with an expert. Your food should bring you joy, and that will happen when you are aligned to it and find it logical.

You probably know these ground rules but let me remind you once again:

1. Leave alcohol and tobacco. On the practical side, keep it under moderate levels.
2. No drugs and narcotics. Sorry, I am not giving any leeway in this.
3. Exercise toh karna pageda (you must do). Even if you are healthy, you must continue with some moderate

exercise. Anything that works for you—gym, strengths, walk, yoga. But keep it moving. On the other side, don't overdo it.
4. Avoid too much of packaged foods or outside food. Fresh home-cooked food is the best.
5. Healthy diet, healthy lifestyle, moderate stress.

Relationship Issues

Infertility management has much to do with mental wellbeing. Your relationships and their impact on you can swing your emotions one way or the other. And I am not talking just about the relationship with your partner but also with your extended family and friends because atleast in India, families do leave a mark on our mental health.

Stay away from relationships that make you unhappy or leave a negative impact. Well! Easier said than done, but this is something you must do because you must focus on resolving infertility and not relationship conflicts at this point in your life.

Not all relations are the same, so not all relations can be treated the same. Here is a quick guide to help you with relationship management based on the type they belong to:

Non-Essential Person Who Impacts You Negatively

A relative, friend or colleague not very close to you, but whenever you do meet, there is some negativity you feel from them. Just distance yourself.

I had this neighbour, let's call her Nosey Aunty. She would often make passing remarks, ' Arrey, how long will you be on your honeymoon? It is time to get a third person in the family.' She even advised that I quit my job to focus on baby-making.

Such random comments would make me sulk.

I tried to avoid her but then she would always find a way to catch me.

Finally, one day I decided to do something about it. I went to her house. She offered me tea. I denied. I looked into her eyes and said in a professional tone, 'Nosey Aunty, I am going through infertility and recently had a miscarriage. I am seeing doctors for treatment. And I really don't like talking about this topic. I would appreciate if you respect this.'

She was startled. She wasn't expecting a hard-hitting conversation like this. I wasn't scared of her anymore. I was free of this nuisance.

Close Family Member Who Impacts You Negatively

This person can be your husband (worst-case scenario), your mother-in-law (most common scenario), your own parents, a very close relative, or family friends. They are the closest people and what they say or do hurt you the most. Thus, the complication.

The option to avoid them completely might not be possible in this case, so we have to manage somehow. They might be truly naive, and their insensitivity is emanating from ignorance about the process. *Communication* is key here. These people love you, but they don't know how to support you. Try to talk, explain, and involve them in the process. Take them for IVF counselling sessions or show them an infertility-themed movie to start the conversation in the right direction. Clearly set the right expectations and a threshold that they shouldn't cross.

If they can't be managed in these ways and you can't avoid them, atleast save yourself from their negativity during the IVF process. Be like the Arjun from the *Mahabharata*, focusing on the eye of the golden fish (conceiving a healthy baby in your case).

The Most Important Person in this Journey, Your Partner

I have seen a supportive husband who cries outside the OT seeing their wife in so much pain, and I have also seen a husband who doesn't even agree to go for a sperm test and puts the complete blame of infertility on the wife.

Let me tell you that infertility is not easy for men either. We will discuss more about male infertility in Chapter 10

I have seen women who begin to ignore the husband completely, engulfed in the anxiety of the treatment. They even stop trying.

Agreed! It is the woman who is getting poked with injections, but the man is feeling vulnerable, too. Walk through this phase as a couple.

1. Go for IVF counselling sessions together.
2. Don't take the relationship or the partner for granted.

3. Spend quality time with each other.
4. Talk about things other than fertility and treatment.
5. Set correct expectations by expressing your true feelings.
6. Do a fun activity together to release the pressure of IVF and to feel the love and joy.
7. Try to understand each other by being compassionate.
8. Be conscious to not hurt your partner.
9. If you felt hurt by anything that your partner said or did, don't keep it in your heart and mull over; instead, tell them.
10. Learn to be resilient in your relationship.

IVF is a tough process and takes a toll emotionally, with constant mood swings, anxiety bouts and stress affecting the marital relationship the most. This is the time to strengthen your bond to smoothly sail through the tough time towards a successful IVF.

If you are unable to cope with relationship stress, don't hesitate to consult a psychologist and get help. Both of you need to stand tall, strong and together. Parenthood is not going to be an easy journey, and this is just the beginning.

Join a Support Group or an Online Community of People Going Through the Same Issues

It helps to be a part of a peer support group where you can connect with couples who have been through similar journeys, share your anxieties, get some practical tips, and get recommendations on doctors/clinics or just bond with no strings attached. When you see so many other couples struggling, you won't feel alone.

The downside of such support groups/online communities is excessive sharing of notes. Yes, this happens more often than we know, and then, that becomes a point of stress. You must ask, share and get notes on each other's treatment or doctor but apply them with a pinch of salt. What works for someone else might not work for you, and second, not everyone will be completely honest while sharing.

'Her IVF costed Rs 1.5 lakhs, then why is my doctor asking for Rs 2.5 lakhs.'

Well! The additional cost might be of donor or blastocyst or freezing. Each case's requirement is different.

'They got successful in IUI but our doctor advised for IVF.'

Again, depends on what your diagnosis is.

Support groups are therapeutic if you don't get swayed by them. Sharing each other's journey gives you strength and hope.

Now that the preparation is all done, let us get the IVF done.

> *'The future belongs to those who believe in the beauty of their dreams.'*
>
> – Eleanor Roosevelt

Stay strong, stay focused!

9
Result Day

THE FOURTEENTH DAY AFTER YOUR EMBRYO TRANSFER FEELS like being back in school after your finals. You are scared, anxious, you've got all your fingers and toes crossed. You're hoping for the best but fearing the worst. Your mind is a mess of emotions.

The Good News

'Congratulations! You are pregnant!'
The words that you have been wanting to hear so desperately, the scene that you had imagined so many times in your head is finally happening. Your HCG blood test report confirms your pregnancy. It is an extremely emotional moment for you. Soak it in.

I remember the moment so clearly, just like it was yesterday. I was sitting on the sofa in the doctor's lobby just outside the report collection counter. The pathologist came over to me and handed me the report, asking me to show it to the doctor. I looked at him searchingly. He reluctantly said, 'The report is positive but show it to the doctor first.'

My heart sank. My mind went blank. I was happy but scared of jinxing it, too. I said to myself, 'Finally, it's happened! But Gitanjali, don't be too happy. Control yourself. You have been pregnant before, but you've not heard the heartbeat. Hold your horses.'

For me, the real joy of pregnancy happened when I heard my baby's heartbeat for the first time. Till then, I couldn't risk being happy.

Never forget that IVF pregnancies are high risk, so the first three months are extremely crucial. After the first trimester, your case is transferred to the gynaecology department and normal pregnancy protocols are followed. However, you can never let your guard down.

'Pain in the Ass' Progesterone Injections

During the first three months, apart from regular medicines like folic acid and multivitamins, you will be prescribed some other medicines as per your individual medical history along with progesterone injections. The main function of progesterone is to maintain the uterine lining to support the growth of the embryo. You have to continue taking progesterone injections for ninety days. As the injection is oil-based and is administered daily, mostly in your bum (intramuscular), it becomes a real *pain in the ass*.

Every morning, before going to office, I would go to the nearby clinic to get the injection. After a month, there was hardly any 'non-sore' space left in my bum to place the injection. The kind Malyali nurse would sympathetically explain in her broken Hindi that she has no option but to inject over the already swollen area. It sure was painful, but the joy of motherhood happily accepts the pain.

Tips to Manage Progesterone Injections:

1. Thankfully, we have two sides of the bum. Alternate the side, thus giving one day's healing time to each side. The catch here is to remember the side, which sadly I used to forget all the time.
2. Massage the area really well after the injection to help the movement of the oil. I always loved this part.
3. A hot massage works like a charm to ease pain. You can apply a heating pad, hot water bottle, hot compress, or vigorously massage the spot. Heat and a massage break down the progesterone, helping it dissolve faster, thus decreasing your pain.
4. Ask your doctor to prescribe a local anaesthesia cream and an anticoagulant gel. Applying these will alleviate the pain.
5. Try to relax the hip and gluteus muscles.
6. You may ask the nurse to administer the injection slowly. This comes from real experience. Initially, I would suffer from a lot of pain when the injections were administered. But when my nurse changed, the pain I felt reduced. The injections were the same, but how it was administered made a world of a difference.

7. Focus on your breathing when the injection is given. Take deep breaths.
8. There's no need to rush after receiving the injection. Take your time. Sometimes, due to rush hour, the nurse might force you to hurry up and leave the room. That's why it's best to get progesterone shots at home. Also, in some cases, women might be advised bed rest.
9. If the pain is unbearable, speak to your doctor who may prescribe progesterone supplements to take orally or vaginally. However, this will depend on your individual medical history. It is best to follow the doctor's advice.

Remember, this too shall pass! On the ninetieth of my progesterone injections, I hugged my nurse tight and partied hard. It was not only the end of a painful routine, but also most importantly, it was time for new beginnings. I was in my second trimester now.

Take prescribed medicines and injections without fail or delay. Some injections need to be administered at a particular time of the day. Make sure that this is done as advised by the doctor. Some injections can be self-administered. If you are scared, then ask your partner to do it.

Listening to Your Baby's Heartbeat

There can be nothing more exciting than hearing your baby's heartbeat for the first time. The baby is finally here. Your doubts are over. Frankly, I could truly celebrate my pregnancy post this milestone.

Don't Let Your Guards Down

IVF pregnancy will mostly be a high-risk pregnancy; so you need to be extra careful and prepared always. I had a minor but scary setback in my second trimester when there was some bleeding and the placenta had come down. I was in my office when the spotting started. I informed my friend, Bhawna, that I am going to the doctor and that something is not right. I called my doctor, who asked me to come right away. The road from my office to the doctor's felt like the longest I had ever taken. Every second felt heavy. Upon reaching, the doctor ran some tests and confirmed that the baby is absolutely fine. I was put on bed rest for two weeks with some medicines.

If not medically complex, IVF pregnancies are surely high on emotions (namely scare).

To Take, or Not to Take Bed Rest—That's the Question

This seems like an encompassing question that keeps popping up all the time. As if taking bed rest is the answer to all our worries of infertility.

'Oh! You are infertile—take bed rest.'

'Oh! Your IVF worked—take bed rest.'

'Oh! Your IVF failed—it was because you didn't take bed rest.'

'You had a miscarriage—you were not on bed rest, that's why it happened.'

Somewhere, I feel it comes from the narrow societal mindset that career women are casual about family, so as an antidote, bed rest becomes symbolic of being careful, cautious, caring, and conscious.

Well! If it partially answers the dilemma of bed rest, I will boldly and happily say that I think I owe it to being working (and not taking bed rest) for having a healthy pregnancy and a full-term delivery when my second IVF succeeded.

Just Ask Yourself A Few Questions to Answer this Dilemma of Bed Rest

1. **Is it your choice or an outside pressure?** Pressure can be subtle or a past guilt (you had a miscarriage earlier where you blamed it for not taking enough bed rest so this time you are driven by that thought of resurrection).
2. **Is taking bed rest advised by the doctor because of some medical reason?** If yes, then don't ever mess with it. In my fourth month, I had spotting and my placenta was low (a common scenario in early pregnancy). My doctors clearly asked me to take bed rest with my feet raised up at 45 degrees for a week. I did exactly that. After a week, I went for an ultrasound, and my placenta was better positioned. I took another week of work from home to be on the safer side.
3. **Is taking bed rest giving you joy?** The baseline goal is to be happy. If taking bed rest is what your body wants, then go for it. Listen to your body.
4. **Does bed rest mean being in bed all the time?** Even if you go for bed rest, I am strongly against the 'practically being chained to the bed' kind of rest. You

are finally pregnant after so many struggles; you must revel in the joy of it every moment.

5. **Are you confusing bed rest with taking care?** Think hard on this one—you can take care of yourself while not being in complete bed rest. I was going to office, but I made sure that the driver was driving slowly and was being careful of potholes, as sudden jerks are not good during pregnancy. I was going to shopping malls but avoiding the rush hours. I was eating out occasionally but was careful of what I pick from the menu. I was going to office but had an open conversation with my boss, Saba Khan—she was the first one in the office to know about my IVF and pregnancy—she was happy to facilitate balance.

Make the right choices. Create the right environment around you. Set a routine. Live a conscious life.

I think these are good enough to sail you through a safe pregnancy.

Try Not to Fall Sick During the Early Stage of IVF Pregnancy

Acidity, nausea, vomiting, bloating, constipation and uneasiness are some of the regular issues during early pregnancy. Compounding with these issues is the fact that you are also taking heavy medicines and injections. The problem with pregnancy is that if you fall sick then you can't take antibiotics since it is harmful for your foetus. So, a good diet and a healthy lifestyle are critical during this period.

Keep Your Mind and Stomach Clear

Stick to the basic rules (as given in Chapter 8)—having healthy home-cooked food, light walking/exercising, taking some natural vitamin D from sunlight, following a balanced lifestyle, sleeping on time and for enough hours, practising meditation—and you should be good to go.

Don't Panic

Recently, I connected with a pregnant woman who was panicking because her baby's heartbeat wasn't detected in the early scan. In another case, the woman experienced spotting post-IVF conception.

There might be hiccups, and that is why the first trimester is a bit tricky. You need to be cautious and careful. Be mindful of any changes in the body. You need to discuss any symptom, however small, with your doctor. In my case, I was experiencing mild constipation for two days and I didn't inform my doctor or take any corrective measures. I thought it would adjust on its own. I was wrong. The next day, while trying to pass stool, I put a little more pressure due to constipation, and within a few hours, I was spotting (there was light bleeding). I was scared. I was prescribed a laxative, some food items were removed from my diet, and

I was put on two weeks' bed rest. Had I connected with the doctor earlier, the situation would have not escalated.

However, try not to panic. Of course, this is easier said than done. All your memories of past failure and struggle will come rushing back into your mind. This is only natural. The golden rule here is to focus on the current moment and resolve it.

Panic won't lead you towards any resolution. If such a scenario crops up, then direct your energy towards solving the problem at hand, and moving on to the next phase of pregnancy.

Don't be Disheartened by Failure

The famous Prime Minister of Britain, Margaret Thatcher, once said, 'You may have to fight a battle more than once to win it.' And nothing could be more applicable to this than failure in the IVF process.

Heena, a thirty-one-year-old budding baker from Gurugram, called me at ten in the night. She had just got the news that her IVF had failed, and she didn't know what to do or think. 'I have failed, I have failed', she kept saying in between sobs.[75]

Another lady, whose real name I don't know, messaged on our Fertility Dost group's (a group for women trying to conceive) chatbot. The message read, 'I will commit suicide.

---

75 Conversation with Heena, a thirty-one-year-old Baker from Gurugram.

This was my third IVF and it, too, has failed. This is the end of the world for me.'

When Purnima (my colleague from Gurugram who was in her thirties when struggling with infertility) had her fourth IVF with twins, it ended in premature delivery and her babies didn't survive even for an hour; she was inconsolable. She couldn't comprehend her own feelings.

Rashi, a twenty-six-year-old homemaker from Lucknow, says:

> When my first IVF failed, I sank into depression. I was lost. My second IVF was all wrong. One, I was not prepared for it. Also, the tests suggested were not right. I felt that during the process the doctors didn't guide me properly and were playing a blame game. I felt I wasn't seeing the right doctor. I was also depressed as I had a tiff with my mother-in-law during my second IVF due to which I also had issues with my husband. This caused immense stress during my second IVF.[76]

'After my failed IVF, I took a long break. I was very exhausted from the treatment. I wanted to take a break from hospitals and medicines and just spend some time with myself. I am now thinking about trying another cycle', says Jaisanavi[77]

---

[76] Interview with Rashi, a twenty-six-year-old homemaker from Lucknow.

[77] Interview with Jaisanavi.

'I was okay most of the times because I knew that I had to do it [IVF]. I didn't think too much. I took it one day at a time! There were ups and downs. But after my second IVF failure, the frustration was high. It was mainly because I was not getting answers', says Simrat Kaur a thirty-five-year-old non-resident Indian (NRI) from Canada who had come to India for her IVF treatment.[78]

These are real life experiences from real women. The one thing that emerges from their stories is, 'You are not alone. Many of you reading this book might have already been through failed IVF. There is no easy way of saying this, but you will have to process the grief and keep moving ahead. And remember, as F. Scott Fitzgerald rightly said, 'Never confuse a single defeat with a final defeat.'

For all other health issues, you are treated as an individual. However, with fertility treatments, you are simultaneously treating two (husband and wife) people, which makes the process more complex. The two of you are intrinsically involved in this process to build a third. Managing three entities is a Herculean task.

The IVF success rate in India is 35 per cent, which means that the failure rate is 65 per cent. In fact, first time IVF failure rate is even higher. As per an Ernst & Young report on IVF in India, a couple usually requires two and a half

---

78 Interview with Simrat Kaur, a thirty-five-year-old NRI from Canada.

IVF cycles (between two and three cycles) on an average to succeed.[79]

No matter how realistic your expectations towards the IVF process is, feelings of loss similar to pregnancy happen because you get attached to the inserted embryos. You have been carefully nurturing yourself as a mother, even though it was for a short period of only two weeks. On hearing the news of conception failure, the grief you feel is real, you stop caring for yourself, and the sudden stopping of hormone injections adds to your woes. It might lead to mood swings as well.

Indu Malik, fertility counsellor and psychologist with Fertility Dost, says that a woman who has undergone an IVF failure goes through the following stages of emotions:

1. **Denial**: 'The report is false, I am pregnant', 'I still feel the embryo inside.'
2. **Anger**: Gets angry with God, doctor, on clinic or oneself—'Why me?'
3. **Bargaining**: 'I should have not eaten this', 'I should have taken better care', etc.
4. **Depression**: The feeling of hopelessness, helplessness and worthlessness is at the peak.
    - *Hopelessness*: 'I will never have a child.'
    - *Helplessness*: 'Nothing is working out in a positive way.'
    - *Worthlessness*: Feeling of inadequacy and inferiority.

---

79 Ernst & Young, 'Call for Action: Expanding IVF treatment in India', July 2015.

5. **Acceptance**: The realization of the IVF cycle failure along with extreme psychological distress.

I will not squander your time by giving more gyaan on how to manage IVF failure emotionally because I know you will take your time, but you will do it, eventually. I would rather focus on some practical aspects which we miss amid the emotional mess we experience when failure hits.

Ask Your Doctor for Reasons behind IVF Failure

When IVF fails, doctors just have a single-line answer: 'Koi baat nahi Madam, fir se kara lena (Don't worry Ma'am! Get the IVF done again).' Kasha (a twenty-seven-year-old who helps in the family business) from Jalandhar, Punjab, repeats her doctor's words. She has been through three failed IVFs, hysteroscopy, laparoscopy, four failed donor egg IVFs, PCOS and tuberculosis, and is now trying to convince her husband to take the surrogacy route.

Understanding why your IVF failed will help you with the closure that you need to process your grief, and will also help you plan the treatment ahead. Sit with your doctor and have an open and honest discussion. I see many couples rushing to their doctor immediately after failure. This conversation then results in an emotionally charged exchange rather than a cool-headed approach. Instead of asking the right questions, you seem to rush towards a conclusion, which can either be too harsh on the doctor (blaming the doctor's incompetence for failure) or be trapped into doing another round of IVF (some doctors may manipulate your vulnerability). Hence, it is a good idea to schedule the meeting with your doctor when you feel better and are ready to talk.

Box 9.1: An Important Tip

> It is also important to get all the documents regarding IVF—the dosage of stimulation, follicles formed, eggs retrieved, embryos formed, number of embryos transferred, grade of embryos transferred, day on which the transfer was done (day three or day five)—all this information in writing. I can't tell you the number of cases I see on a daily basis where clinics withhold this information or simply communicate to patients verbally. This poses a challenge if you decide to change clinics for the next round of IVF. The next doctor needs to know everything about your medical history so that they don't have to start from ground zero.

Source: Created by the author.

Hemlata, in her early thirties, pursing her PhD from Kolkata, recounts that when her IVF failed at clinic A (a renowned chain of IVF clinics), she decided to consult a new doctor. Soon, she realized that some information about her previous IVF was missing, which was critical for the new doctor to even give a proper second opinion. When she contacted clinic A, they quoted policy restrictions and said that they only give a certain amount of information. They also offered a good discount if she gets her next IVF done at their clinic. Hemlata was persistent. It took her almost three months, several rounds to the clinic, emails to senior management, when they finally relented, and that too, 'on a special request basis', to hand over her file.

It is also important to listen and calmly try to understand what the doctor has to say. You can't put the doctor in 'Aap Ki Adalat' (a mock courtroom in an Indian TV show of the same name) and shoot out hateful questions and statements even if you are extremely upset. It is quite possible that the doctor won't have a concrete answer as to why your IVF failed. However, at the same time, don't accept a response which is vague, like, 'It happens.' A doctor's sincerity will be evident in how they assist you in this crucial phase.

Dr Sulbha (an IVF specialist in Mumbai) once said, 'I give more time to couples who have had a failed IVF because they had trusted me, and it is my duty to explain to them what went wrong. I know they are going through a very tough phase of life. I feel bad for them, especially because sometimes even I don't have answers to why the IVF failed. At this point, my compassion is the best I can offer them.'

Both the patient and the doctor must reach out to each other with trust, integrity and compassion. The goal of this exercise is to understand what went wrong in the hope of finding answers that lead us to the right treatment path.

Dr Parul, a senior IVF expert, Delhi, says that when IVF fails, she falls back on the following checklist:

1. Make sure to engage a fertility counsellor in the conversation.
2. Transparently discuss the reasons that led to the failure.
3. Discuss how we can improve the outcome from here onwards.
4. Give examples of patients with similar cases and the stages of failure in their fertility journeys. They even do a 'circle of hope' by bringing patients together to share their journeys in a safe space. This provides reassurance and helps them process the grief.

She strongly emphasizes that there is no point in deliberating too much on what went wrong because unfortunately, they often don't have answers about failed cases because they go ahead with IVF only when all the markers look good.

Dr Sonia Malik, a senior IVF consultant, New Delhi, says, 'When we focus on fact-finding, when we as doctors are ready with an action list to find out what went wrong and talk to the patient transparently, then there is no reason as to why they will mistrust or not cooperate.'[80]

According to Dr Munjaal Kapadia, an IVF expert, Mumbai, who is himself a proud IVF father, every IVF failure is equally devastating for him. 'We don't blankly

---

80 Interview with Dr Sonia Malik, a senior IVF consultant, New Delhi.

say to the patient, "Haan, sab accha hai." We ensure that there is transparency, involvement and communication. These are the three most important pillars to efficiently managing an IVF patient. Don't paint a rosy picture. Keep it real. I repeatedly tell a couple, 'Even though you have the best eggs, best embryos, best lining, that doesn't mean it will automatically translate into a success. We will try our best, but in IVF there are multiple factors.'[81] The idea is to prepare the couple well and set realistic expectations. There are no 100per cent results.

Dr Munjaal candidly shares that those IVF cases where there is a conception, but the pregnancy terminates early, are the most difficult cases to handle. They must be extremely gentle and compassionate with such couples. 'As doctors, we can't let them give up on their dreams of having a baby due to frustration with the treatment', he says.[82]

Investigate and Find the Root Cause

No one knows your body better than you; no one wants the baby as much as you do. In fact, by now, you have become half a doctor yourself and are quite comfortable with fertility-medico jargon.

When my first IVF failed, I had this one racing thought that wouldn't let me rest—'What went wrong?' Post the initial stress phase, when I was finally able to collect myself, I sat

---

81 Interview with Dr Munjaal Kapadia, an IVF expert, Mumbai.
82 Ibid.

with my thick medical file where carefully and chronologically all the medical documents like tests reports, diagnosis, prescriptions, injection schedules, hospital admissions, etc., were punched together. I went through them thoroughly, scanning each paper, recalling each conversation with the doctor. I had changed somewhere between six to eight doctors during my fertility journey, and not to mention a few where I simply went for a second opinion consultation. My gut feeling said that I had missed something. After a few days of this exercise, I recalled this Christian doctor who I was consulting when my third miscarriage happened, and he had hinted towards a genetic issue, which at that time I had completely ignored due to the emotional rollercoaster that I was going through. I immediately booked a consultation with a genetic counsellor. Further treatment path correction came from this one revelation.

> *It is not a lost opportunity, it is a lesson ...*
> *Find strength in your sorrows.*

A lot of the times, doctors can't give you individual attention. At the end of the day, it is just a job for them and you, yet another case. Also, you might have changed a few doctors during the journey and now you have a huge pile of papers with clashing opinions, repeated tests, and too much of going back and forth. It is natural to lose track and get confused. Take a step back, take a relook at all the medical documents, and look for gaps, which can be anything for you: stress, lack of preparatory time, missed advanced test, a diagnosis you overlooked earlier because it wasn't the easier choice, or a messed-up environment. Figure them out and plug them in before jumping into the next phase of treatment after the failure.

Taking it to the Next Level

A failed IVF is a major roadblock in your fertility journey because not only have you invested money in it, but you are also stressed to a breaking point. At this stage, most doctors usually suggest another round of IVF and some advanced tests.

Rujeta, a thirty-seven-year-old banker from Gurgaon, had just been through her first IVF failure. Her doctor suggested one more round of IVF with this logic: 'Sometimes it doesn't work out in the first attempt.' I asked Rujeta to ask her doctor, specifically about what treatment protocol they were suggesting for the next round of IVF. It is no point doing the same protocol that they had followed last time. Usually, the doctors will suggest an advanced test (to dig deeper into the reason behind the failure) or an advanced protocol (like frozen embryo transfer, donor IVF cycle, ICSI, and the like) or a corrective procedure (like plasma therapy or preimplantation genetic diagnosis [PGD], and the like) to increase chances of success. Talk about your options with your doctor.

Think about it like this: What do you do if you fail an academic exam? You plan to study or prepare for it differently, right? You study harder, you get new reading material, or you change your study routine. You tweak something. The same formula applies when it comes to failed IVFs.

Talk to your doctor. If they are not able to convince you logically, then change your doctor or get a second opinion. Also, be wary of doctors who place too much emphasis on finding faults with your previous doctor in a bid to prove their superiority. A good approach is to concentrate on what they plan to do next and how.

Dr Munjaal says, 'Instead of snubbing the patient for asking questions inspired by Googling, I give them credible articles and websites to read and research, prepare their questions for discussion before getting into the treatment.'[83]

Talk to an IVF counsellor (not the ones who sit at IVF clinics, who for obvious reasons can't be critical of their doctors) and get neutral advice.

Here are some things to think about:

1. You may want to consider if a different type of IVF is better suited for you.

Maybe an egg donor IVF cycle was better suited to you, but you were not able to take that call due to moral stigmas. Now is the time to let go of all prejudices and think clearly. The type of IVF you choose is an important factor in reaching the final goal. Spend time chewing on this before making this decision. Research, ask around, take a second opinion,

---

[83] Interview with Dr Munjaal.

think with an open mind, and talk to people who have been through IVF. Take your time but take a wise decision.

2. Could an advanced test help you pinpoint and alleviate the problem area?

Couples in non-metropolitan cities might not be able to access advanced tests or techniques that have the potential to provide solutions for infertility. But don't let that stop you from asking your doctors about these tests. If they don't have it in their clinic, then the chances are that they will undermine its importance. These tests are:

- ERA test.
- PGD.
- Genetic counselling.

These are expensive, so you must be careful before opting for them. These add-on tests and procedures are not meant for everyone, and their success depends on your specific medical condition. Think hard on the following questions:

- Do you really need them?
- Do they promise to significantly increase your success chances?
- Is it worth taking that chance?
- Do they have any side effects?

3. Did you miss out on alternative methodologies to support your IVF?

I can never emphasize enough the importance of alternative methodologies (see Chapter 8), which are sadly due to low marketing strength is underrated and unacknowledged. See Chapter 8, which is dedicated to alternative methodologies.

4. Have you handled your subtle and emotional issues?

Suman Kaur, a thirty-two-year-old accountant from Punjab, had just started her IVF cycle when her father-in-law fell sick and was hospitalized. Needless to say, due to this stressful situation, her IVF cycle failed. Apart from working on your emotional wellbeing, you also need to ensure that the environment around you is conducive to your fertility journey. In Suman's case, the situation was not under her control, but in most of the cases, it can be. Are you doing enough to create that environment?

Take a Break

Ideally, there should be a six-month gap between two IVF cycles. Some clinics might push you into invasive tests and treatments from the very next month after your failed IVF. This might not be the best thing to do. Your mind and body can only take so much. You need a break to take your mind completely off the treatment. This will help you stabilize and think clearly.

Women, Don't Blame Your Partner; Men, Don't Let Your Partner Sink

Fatima is a thirty-three-year-old sales executive from Vadodara. An educated and independent woman who comes from a conservative family, says:

> With so many ups and downs and back-to-back IVF failures, my stress and anxiety levels were at their peak. I had a tough time with my husband, and my marriage was about to fall apart. I did blame my partner many a times. I also had a problem with my peers. There was a lot of societal indifference especially from people who already had children and this hurts a lot.[84]

This is the most common reaction post IVF failure. The husband becomes the punching bag. What they forget is that although men might not be expressive, infertility is exhaustive for them, too. They are also new to this and have no clue on how to handle it. Men, mostly caught between an IVF failure and an inconsolable wife, tend to retract into their shells.

---

84 Interview with Fatima, a thirty-three-year-old sales executive from Vadodara.

It is a dismal life situation where both of you are heartbroken, clueless and pessimistic about the future. It is absolutely normal to have a sinking feeling. Just don't hide your emotions. Talk to each other, vent out the grief (not on each other), and the best way to break this cycle of grief is to start planning for the path ahead, focusing all your energies there.

Don't Put a Timeline to Life

It is good to have a roadmap for your pregnancy journey, but don't put strict timelines on milestones like career and family. Most women have a mental timeline—career at twenty-eight, marriage by thirty years and a kid by thirty-two years! Majja ni life! Don't put too much pressure on yourself, thinking that time is slipping away. I was thirty-three when I became a mother. I found my peace in the thought that if I were to have two kids, then I would have planned the first baby at around twenty-five to twenty-seven years and the second one after a gap of five years. With my situation of infertility, I had my first child at thirty-three, which was still in the broader timeline given to the conception stage of life, and I tweaked it a bit by forgoing the plan of a second baby. To conclude, I was not late for motherhood, right? I now have one kid, which in retrospect works so much better for me.

Sometimes, a change of perspective can make the burden much lighter to bear.

Box 9.2: Coping ideas

- Identify, accept and acknowledge your emotions.
- Grieve the failure and loss properly. Don't let anybody tell you otherwise or push you if you aren't ready.
- Grieve, but not alone. Take your partner along. It is not 'I' who is grieving but 'we', and this will make the burden so much lighter and the hope stronger.
- Practise self-love.
- Seek professional help if you can't break the pattern within a stipulated time.
- Don't isolate yourself completely. It is natural to get into your shell, but try to go out with whoever you are comfortable with.

Source: Created by the author.

10

Male Infertility
The Elephant in the Room

'Like men, sperm are also taken for granted. Among the millions of sperm, only one needs to do the job and serve masculinity.
As many as 2 per cent of all men will show below average sperm quality.' [85]

THIS IS THE SHOCKING TRUTH. AND YET, MALE INFERTILITY is discussed under wraps and is directly connected to male ego where low sperm count is wrongly understood as being less of a man.

---

85 N. Kumar and A.K. Singh, 'Trends of Male Infertility, an Important Cause of Infertility: A Review of Literature', *Journal of Human Reproductive Sciences* 8, no. 4 (2015), pp. 191–96, available at https://www.ncbi.nlm.nih.gov/pmc/articles/PMC4691969/.

Male Infertility

'Kya hua abhi tak baccha nahi hua, bahu ka test karwaya kya? [Your daughter-in-law didn't conceive yet? What happened? Did you get her tested?]'

This is the most common statement I've heard when it comes to couples who are having trouble conceiving. Society invariably assumes that the fault lies with the woman. But we need to point the lens at both men and women because it takes two to tango, and two to make a baby.

Most men are all about numbers. So, let's begin with numbers:

1. 40 per cent of reported infertility cases are related to male causes, while 40 per cent have female causes,
2. 20 per cent of infertility cases have mixed issues from both men and women.[86]
3. For Indian couples seeking treatment, the male factor is the cause in approximately 23 per cent cases.[87]

These statistics clearly show that men are equally responsible for infertility. And yet, it is usually women who bear its

---

[86] B.J. Sadock and V.A. Sadock, 'Kaplan and Sadock's Synopsis of Psychiatry', *Indian Journal of Psychiatry* 51, no. 4 (2009), pp. 872–74, Behavioural Sciences/Clinical Psychiatry, Tenth Edition.

[87] A.H. Zargar, A.I. Wani, S.R. Masoodi, B.A. Laway and M. Salahuddin, 'Epidemiologic and Etiologic Aspects of Primary Infertility in the Kashmir Region of India', *Fertility and Sterility* 68, no. 4 (1997), pp. 637–43, available at https://www.fertstert.org/article/S0015-0282(97)00269-0/pdf.

brunt. Aiza vociferously expresses that people should stop blaming the female every time:

> The first thing society does is point at a female. They never blame the male. What they don't understand is that the couple is a team. It's not just one person to be blamed. And people should become more open towards the accomplishments of female. The only thing we women require is respect from society and the husband. And, when we don't get that our world falls apart.[88]

What Can Go Wrong?

Before we dive into the nitty-gritties of male infertility, there is an interesting perspective that I'd like to share with you.

- ☑ **The good thing** (yes, there is a good thing, too!) about male infertility is that men just need to go through one test—the sperm test. Better still is that sperm tests are not invasive, they are easy can be diagnosed using them, and diagnosis happens in 80–90 per cent of the cases. In female infertility, however, a woman has to undergo many diagnostic tests, which are mostly invasive and inconclusive. Blame it on the lack of research on male infertility or how men have it easy, but the fact is that male infertility is much easier to diagnose when compared to female infertility.

---

88 Interview with Aiza.

☒ **The problem**, however, is that while it is easy to diagnose male infertility through one test, it is extremely difficult for them to take that test, owing to the huge social taboo which has construed the idea of masculinity. Not to overtly generalize, but I would put a disclaimer that there are many men who are proactive, and in fact, offer to get their test done before beginning with their female partners' tests. And then, there are men who keep delaying the treatment because they are not ready to go for the test.

On that note, let us quickly understand the basic infertility triggers for men.

Causes of Male Infertility

Age

Age matters in male infertility, too, but the intensity of the impact is much lower than what it is in female infertility. So, men can relax a bit on this age parameter. Male fertility begins to decline after forty years (though it is an insignificant drop) with a decline in testosterone levels and more after the fifty-five year mark.[89]

---

89 I.D. Harris, C. Fronczak, L. Roth and R.B. Meacham, 'Fertility and the Aging Male', *Reviews in Urology* 13, no. 4 (2011), pp. e184–90, available at https://www.ncbi.nlm.nih.gov/pmc/articles/PMC3253726/.

Psychosexual Issues

Psychosexual issues are when you are fine physically, but due to some emotional and psychological barriers, you are unable to perform sexual activity. I recently came across a couple who were advised IVF; however, on deeper investigation, it turned out that they were not consummating their marriage (having sex) properly, as the male partner had psychosexual issues. With a few sessions with the psychologist, conception happened naturally.

Psychosexual issues are the most common cause of erectile dysfunction. Dr Sujal Torgil Patil, an Ayurvedic doctor and fertility consultant practising in Goa, says,

> In case of erectile dysfunction, the problem may not be solved by going for a specific sex position and needs to have complete integrated approach which can improve the chances of conception. The position that is comfortable for both the partners, wherein the blood flows into the penile area is better and the muscles involved perform better, is ideally the best. The emotional quotient matters more that the physical quotient here.[90]

If such is the case, meet a psychologist and revive your marital relations and conception chances.

---

90 Interview with Dr Sujal Torgil Patel, Ayurvedic doctor and fertility consultant, Goa.

Hormone Imbalance

Yes, men, too, have hormonal issues which impact their fertility. Testosterone, luteinizing hormone (LH), FSH, TSH, oestrogen and prolactin are the key that impact male fertility. FSH hormone stimulates the production of sperms while testosterone has direct impact on sex drive and erectile function.

Be mindful of signs like weight gain, hair fall and lower libido, as they can be indicative of hormonal imbalance.

Oxidative Stress

Spermatozoa membranes that constitute a sperm are sensitive to oxygen-induced damage. In a normal situation, the antioxidants will counterbalance the negative impact of the reactive oxygen species (ROS), but when antioxidants in the body are lower (which creates imbalance), it lets the ROS damage the sperms, and this process is known as oxidative stress, the most common factor causing deterioration of sperms in men.[91] Basically, when oxidants outnumber the antioxidants, oxidative stress occurs.

$$\text{Oxidants} = \text{Antioxidant} \text{-----} \text{Normal Sperm Conditions}$$

---

91 S.C. Sikka, 'Oxidative Stress and Role of Antioxidants in Normal and Abnormal Sperm Function', *Frontiers in Bioscience* 1 (1996), pp. e78–86, available at https://www.imrpress.com/journal/FBL/1/5/10.2741/A146.

Oxidants More = Antioxidants Less = Oxidative Stress -------Abnormal Sperm Conditions

Prolonged oxidative stress is even known to cause structural DNA damage.[92] There are stages of damage that oxidative stress can cause, starting from a simple loss of sperm membrane, reduced sperm motility, often escalating to DNA damage.

Oxidative stress happens due to lifestyle issues like stress, smoking, high body mass index (BMI) and overheating of the area around the scrotum. It is for this reason that keeping the laptop or mobile devices close to genital organs, wearing tight undergarments, and taking excessively hot showers is not advised for men.

Oral antioxidant medicines are prescribed. Usually, with an antioxidant-rich diet and a conscious lifestyle along with antioxidants and antibiotic medicines, there is significant improvement in overall sperm quality.

Box 10.1: Male Fertility Recommended Diet

> Vitamin C protects from DNA damage. Wheatgrass juice (WGJ) contains a high concentration of vitamin C, useful for the detoxification and filtration of the blood, builds immunity, boosts fertility, and increases

---

[92] A.T. Alahmar, 'Role of Oxidative Stress in Male Infertility: An Updated Review', *Journal of Human Reproductive Sciences* 12, no. 1 (2019), pp. 4–18, available at https://www.ncbi.nlm.nih.gov/pmc/articles/PMC6472207/.

sexual desire because of the high magnesium content in the phytochemical pigment (chlorophyll), which boosts the production of the enzymes that restores sex steroids.

Vitamin E protects the cell membranes. Take it as a supplement or through the intake of food items like seafood, cheese and eggs.

Vitamin B9 (folic acid) is essential for DNA metabolism and deficiency of this vitamin can cause genetic issues of the embryo or recurrent miscarriages. B9 is abundantly found in green leafy vegetables, liver, milk and eggs.

Lycopene, found in tomatoes improves sperm count and concentration.

Carnitines improve sperm quality, and 75 per cent of carnitines can be obtained from food items like dairy products, chicken, red meat and fish.

Q-10 Coenzyme (CoQ, CoQ10) is known to protect the sperm cell membrane. Take it as a nutritional supplement and add food items like meat, fish, vegetable oils, nuts, vegetables, fruits, cereals and dairy products in your diet.

Zinc improves progressive sperm motility and sperm concentration. Zinc is found in nuts, legumes, seafood, yogurt, fish and milk.

Selenium suppresses testicular toxicity and is found in garlic, onion, broccoli and fish.

Source: E. Torres-Arce, B. Vizmanos, N. Babio, F. Marquez-Sandoval and A. Salas Huetos, 'Dietary Antioxidants in the

Treatment of Male Infertility: Counteracting Oxidative Stress', *Biology (Basel)* 10, no. 3 (2021), pp. 241, available at https://www.ncbi.nlm.nih.gov/pmc/articles/PMC8003818/.

Infections and Inflammations

Owing to the vagaries of modern-day life, infections and inflammations are quite common. Pollution, stress and stretched lifestyles have become an integral part of our life. Usually, doctors prescribe antioxidants, antibiotics and nutraceutical medicines (as the case requires) on a preventive basis as a blanket cover when you start with fertility treatments. After consulting your doctor, you can also consider adding multivitamins to build your immunity. Being physically active is recommended. Consider playing a sport, going to the gym, doing yoga, or any similar activity.

Diabetes

High glucose levels can also cause infertility in men by increasing the rate of hypogonadism, which is a condition when the body produces less than normal and required levels of testosterone hormone, which is an essential male hormone.

The DNA of the sperm may be damaged due to high glucose levels, leading to the natural death of the sperm, thereby making it difficult for the spouse to become pregnant. Diabetes can also lower sexual drive by lowering testosterone levels.

Retrograde ejaculation is another major side effect of diabetes. Due to retrograde ejaculation, men are unable to perform a full-fledged ejaculation of sperm, which results in the semen going back into the bladder instead of being ejaculated normally during sex. In these cases, although the sperm count may look healthy, the ejaculated sperm count is lower, thus reducing chances of impregnation.

Due to high glucose levels, nerves and blood vessels can't be controlled properly because of which leads to erectile dysfunction, and may further lead to impotence.

Common Issues with Sperm Causing Male Infertility

Sperm count

Recent studies have shown that atleast 2 per cent of all men have sperm-related issues like low sperm count, poor sperm motility and/or abnormal shape.[93]

First, this is not a scary scenario. A low sperm count is a fairly common problem, and it can also be treated easily. A normal sperm count is in the range of 15 million sperm to more than 200 million sperm per millilitre (mL) of semen. Anything less than 15 million sperm per millilitre is considered to be a low sperm count.

---

93 Kumar and Singh, 'Trends of Male Infertility.'

Practically, you will only need one sperm to impregnate, but it is important that the sperm count is healthy for an increased chance of conception. That's why many a times, even if the sperm count is in range but on the lower side, doctors will suggest improving it further.

Having a low sperm count is also known as oligospermia in more medical terms (so don't get stressed out if the doctor says you have oligospermia), wherein:

- Mild oligospermia is 10–15 million sperm/mL.
- Moderate oligospermia is 5–10 million sperm/mL.
- Severe oligospermia is diagnosed when the sperm count falls between 0 and 5 million sperm/mL.

A low sperm count might happen due to stress, underlying infections and inflammations, high blood pressure (BP) and cholesterol levels, obesity, and a bad lifestyle. You will be prescribed some medicines, and asked to keep moderate lifestyle, control habits like smoking and drinking, and devise ways to reduce daily stress. Basically, get some fresh air!

You can also try alternative therapies like yoga, meditation, Ayurveda and naturopathy to improve your sperm count. Some of the yoga asanas that are beneficial for male fertility are Bhastrika Pranayama, Sethubandh Asana, Dhanur Asana, Ashwani Mudra, Hal Asana and Nadi Shodhan Pranayama.

Include physical activity in your routine to tackle office stress. Plan a break and spend some quality time with your loved ones.

Box 10.2: Fact Check[94]

> According to a research, chain smoking and regular consumption of alcohol reduces the sperm count by 13–17 per cent. It was also observed that within thirty days of giving up on smoking, the sperm parameters were reversed for good. Try quitting smoking during the pre-conception phase.
>
> Fighting infertility can be challenging as a couple, and this is your chance to step up to share the burden and experience the journey together.

Source: Created by the author.

Sperm Motility

Sperm motility is a condition when the sperm are not moving or swimming adequately. This is important to achieve pregnancy because the sperm are supposed to swim up to the egg. If the sperm are slower than normal or they do not swim properly, then it is a major roadblock for natural conception. Poor sperm motility is also known as asthenozoospermia.

In normal conditions, at least 40 per cent of ejaculated sperm are expected to be motile and reach the destination aka the egg.

---

94 J.R. Kovac, A. Khanna and L.I. Lipshultz, 'The Effects of Cigarette Smoking on Male Fertility', *Postgraduate Medical Journal* 127, no. 3 (2015), pp. 338–41, available at https://www.tandfonline.com/doi/full/10.1080/00325481.2015.1015928.

The range of sperm motility is:

- Normal: 20 million.
- Poor: Lower than 5 million is poor sperm motility.
- Severe: Less than 1 million is severe poor sperm motility.

Sperm motility and morphology are closely linked. If a sperm is not formed properly then it leads to lower motility. Other reasons of bad motility are excessive smoking, issues with male reproductive tract, exposure to chemical or being in an occupation that is physically hazardous.

Sperm Morphology

A sperm has two parts: a head and a tail. A normal sperm will have an oval head and a long tail. Misshapen sperms can have a giant head, short head, double head, double tail, and thickened mid-piece or similar incongruities.

Firstly, getting pregnant with malformed sperm is a problem and secondly, if pregnancy happens then either it ends in a genetic issue or midterm pregnancy loss. Male infertility is based on a combination of all the three important factors of sperm—count, motility, and morphology.

Azoospermia

Azoospermia is a condition when there is either no sperm at all or extremely few sperm in the semen. As per statistics,

1 per cent of male infertility cases can be attributed to azoospermia.[95] Azoospermia can happen due to infections in childhood, genetic factors, physical abnormalities, hormonal disorder, testicular damage, and failure or swelling of blood vessels around the testes.

The solution to this problem is surgical and invasive. Testicular sperm extraction-intracytoplasmic sperm injection (TESE-ICSI) involves the harvesting of sperm from the testicles and is a recommended solution to achieve pregnancy when men are diagnosed with azoospermia. Another option, although aggressive, is the use of donor sperms.

Varicocele

Varicocele is one of the most common conditions that causes male infertility, affecting 15–20 per cent of all men and about 40 per cent of men suffering from infertility.[96] In this condition, the veins around the scrotum dilate and enlarge due to the compression of a vein, causing pain or swelling around the testicular area in some cases. However, in most men, there might not be any significant symptoms or pain, and this makes varicocele even more difficult to diagnose.

---

95 'Azoospermia', Health, Johns Hopkins Medicine, available at https://www.hopkinsmedicine.org/health/conditions-and-diseases/azoospermia.

96 S.W. Leslie, S. Husain and L.E. Siref, *Varicocele*, StatPearls, 27 May 2022, available at https://www.ncbi.nlm.nih.gov/books/NBK448113/.

This testicular damage impacts testosterone levels and is known to damage the sperm in terms of count, shape and motility (the ability to move). Usually, during infertility diagnosis when the sperm test report is extremely abysmal and the patient is not responding to regular treatment protocol, then the doctor would incidentally suspect varicocele. Colour flow doppler test or thermal imaging is suggested to diagnose the severity of varicocele.

The Two Major Tests

The Semen Analysis Test

Semen analysis is the single most important test for diagnosing male infertility. You might be asked to do some additional advanced tests if any anomalies are diagnosed in basic semen analysis test (also popularly known as the sperm test).

If the sperm analysis is poor, it is indicative of chromosomal abnormality and further investigation with advanced tests is required. Some additional tests that you might be asked to undergo are serum FSH, scrotal doppler and genetic tests, serum LH, prolactin and testosterone levels.

The DFI Test

If the sperms are looking good on the outside but are still making bad embryos, then it can be a case of DNA fragmentation, which is the separation or breaking of DNA strands into pieces. This is usually ascertained after an IVF failure or in cases of recurrent miscarriages and unexplained infertility. To rule out this condition, an advanced test called the DFI is conducted.

Higher DFI indicates that the sperm have more DNA damage.

Treatment Options

Once the sperm issues are managed either by medicines to improve overall sperm health or testicular sperm extraction (TESE) for azoospermia cases or magnetic-activated cell sorting (MACS) for DNA fragmentation, and thereafter, the ART protocol is followed, keeping in mind the female partner's issues and corrections required.

Microscopic Testicular Sperm Extraction (MicroTESE) — Surgical Sperm Retrieval

This is the latest technology in infertility treatment that allows for the targeted removal of sperm from the testicles. While traditional methods like testicular biopsy, fine needle aspiration cytology (FNAC), etc., have poor success rates in finding sperm once azoospermia is confirmed in the semen analysis, couples find hope in MicroTESE. If there is nil sperm, as per the sperm test, but the advanced hormone test shows that there might be a few sperm, which will, however, require a strong nudge, and only then sperm can be removed directly from the testes using a tiny needle.

Sperm retrieval rates are high with minimum testicular trauma. This is a minor surgical procedure done under general anaesthesia and takes over three to four hours to complete. Search for sperm is done under a twenty-five times strong microscope. Sperms found are then used for ICSI-IVF.

MACS — To Sieve Out Normal Sperm

To rectify the issue of sperm fragmentation, MACS is suggested. It is an advanced procedure that can separate sperm with high DNA fragmentation from regular ones. Then, the normal sperms are used for IUI or ICSI-IVF to achieve pregnancy success.

Embolization or Varicocelectomy

For men with varicocele condition severely impacting their fertility, the embolization process is carried out. The purpose is to divert the blood from the enlarged vein. This is done by aspirating the vein with a small needle and inserting coil or a liquid to divert the blood flow. For most men, an increase in sperm count and quality is seen after the surgery.

In more serious cases of varicocele, varicocelectomy surgery is performed, where the blood supply to the affected vein is cut off completely. This is usually the second option and is recommended when embolization doesn't work or can't be performed due to some anatomical reason (the vein being inaccessible or a structural issue).

Other Treatment Options

IUI

This is a simple and inexpensive process in which the semen is washed in the lab before it is inserted into the woman's uterus. This improves the quality of the semen, and therefore, the chances of fertilization are quite high.

IVF-ICSI

For low- and poor-quality sperms, IVF done using ICSI methodology improves success rates. In this procedure, good quality sperms are selected using a sophisticated procedure leaving the bad ones out. There is no conclusive research that ICSI increases the conception chances more than a regular IVF.[97] Still, in India, most clinics routinely do ICSI even when sperm report is not severely poor. The cost of ICSI is usually higher than a normal IVF cycle, approximately around Rs 2 lakhs. Choose ICSI only if it is necessary in your particular case and not simply because the clinic says, 'It increases your success chances.' Ask them how, and by how much.

---

97 M. Eftekhar, F. Mohammadian, F. Yousefnejad, B. Molaei and A. Aflatoonian, 'Comparison of Conventional IVF Versus ICSI in Non-male Factor, Normresponder Patients', *Iranian Journal of Reproductive Medicine* 10, no. 2 (2012), pp. 131–36, available at https://www.ncbi.nlm.nih.gov/pmc/articles/PMC4163275/#:~:text=We%20found%20the%20superiority%20of,male%20factor%20subfertility%20(8).

Donor Sperms

Needless to say, if none of the above works, opting for donor sperm is a great way to enjoy parenthood. There are sperm banks that help donors. However, in India, male ego and the patriarchal mindset is a big challenge that prohibits this treatment process. The truth is that babies conceived using donor sperms are biologically yours because the egg is your wife's and the baby grows inside her body. So, the child is every cent yours. It is just the regressive mindset that needs to go! If you are stuck in a situation like this, then don't think twice, do away with your false ideas and ego and enjoy parenthood.

Dr Munjaal says that it is not like a *Vicky Donor* kind of a scenario where a random college guy donates sperms in exchange for money. Of course, nobody enjoys a donor sperm conversation and it is always shocking for the couple. You can't bully them to make this decision. It is natural for them to do a back and forth. It takes time for them to come around to this decision. 'I tell the husband—"put yourself in your wife's shoes. Suppose she had issues with her egg, and we suggested opting for donor eggs, then wouldn't you have gone ahead with it? At least it gives you a fair chance at parenthood".'[98]

Unexplained Male Infertility

In 40–75 per cent of infertile men, there is no demonstrated cause.[99] Often, sperm issues can be idiopathic owing to

---

98   Interview with Dr Munjaal.

99   G.R. Dohle, G.M. Colpi, T.B. Hargreave, G.K. Papp, A. Jungwirth, W. Weidner, EAU Working Group on Male Infertility,

lifestyle and environmental issues. This means that the sperm analysis report can be off track slightly and there is no identified cause for it. This happens due to recent obesity, work stress, a sedentary lifestyle, high BP, high cholesterol, smoking or alcohol intake increase, bad sleep cycle, and the like.

Obesity/being overweight may result in hypogonadism, increased scrotal temperatures, impaired spermatogenesis, decreased sperm concentration and motility, and increased sperm DNA damage.[100]

The good news, however, is that these factors are totally in our control. Small life alterations and tweaks, a bit of moderation, and being self-conscious can help you sail through these tough times. I have already spoken about alternative and holistic approaches in Chapter 8. Experiment and see what works best for you. The only promise you've got to make is to proactively do something about it because you know there is someone else sailing with you in this suffering, desperate to reach the shore.

'EAU Guidelines of Male Infertility', European Urology 48, no. 5 (2005), pp. 703–11, available at https://pubmed.ncbi.nlm.nih.gov/16005562/.

100 S.S. Kasturi, J. Tannir and R.E. Brannigan, 'The Metabolic Syndrome and Male Infertility', *Journal of Andrology* 29, no. 3 (2013), pp. 251–59, available at https://onlinelibrary.wiley.com/doi/full/10.2164/jandrol.107.003731.

Issues of Mind Management

Acceptance

The primary problem with male infertility is related to its acceptance. Some men find even going for a sperm test a question on their masculinity, leading to marital conflicts and derailment of the treatment process. On the other hand, some men will proactively go for the test with an underlying confidence that there can be nothing wrong with them as they are sexually active and are the so-called 'alpha men'. However, the problem begins when the report is not so good as the sperm report, in their mind, equals to a report card of 'being a man' and they think they have failed it.

It is true that women also find it difficult to accept infertility, but owing to social conditioning, if the sole burden of infertility falls on men, it becomes a huge emotional roadblock, hampering the course of treatment.

Since birth, men have been conditioned to be strong, to not cry; they have been pampered as complete human beings on whom the family and society depends; so, when infertility strikes at the core of their basic nature and belief, acceptance is no easy task. And we can't solely blame men for being hardliners for it has been ing rained in them since a young age. Rethinking these stereotypes in a society that believes in masculinity requires a lot of inner engineering and grit.

Based on his experience, Dr Munjaal says that men are now more receptive to these tests especially in urban-centric areas. He says,

> Men are not resistant. It is simply a side-effect of their insecurity. As doctors and counsellors, if we try to talk to them with compassion and tell them that this is not a big deal and that it is treatable then with time they come around. However, if they are from parts of country where male egos are historically accentuated by social patriarchy then it is much trickier.[101]

The solution to infertility lies in moving ahead on the right treatment path. Wasting too much time deliberating on social conditioning or establishing blame eventually harms both of you.

Of course, everyone needs time to accept the shock of infertility. Men, too. If you are taking more time stuck in this phase due to social conditioning, an unforgiving family, or are suffering from anxiety, it is best to seek help. You can't afford to waste too much time deliberating at this stage. You must understand that time and age play a pivotal role in the success of fertility treatments. Having said that, you can't go into the treatment with a messed-up mind. It is best to seek help of a professional counsellor or join a support group.

---

101 Interview with Dr Munjaal.

Men Don't Talk

Deepan, a thirty-three-year-old IT professional and budding blogger, currently living in the US for a project, says:

> I have many male friends with whom I have bonded since college hostel days talking about insecurities ranging from financial, parents and yes even relationship but why was it so hard to make it happen again over infertility?
>
> I remember looking at a giant corkboard with heart shaped messages from hundreds of infertile women reaching out to comfort other women feeling scared or anxious about the process. Unfortunately, none of the messages or groups was about men or talked about their issues. I knew what the real issue was—*the silence*.[102]

Talking, venting and crying won't come to men naturally. And that's absolutely okay. I think a wife can be the best friend to a husband, especially for this part of life's journey. Women must be proactive in creating a safe and non-judgemental space for men to emote and releive their anxiety because then, together, you both can give the best to the treatment. Trust me, there are so many decisions to be made during one's fertility journey that it becomes imperative for a couple to work together as a team to navigate it successfully.

---

[102] Interview with Deepan, a thirty-three-year-old IT professional, temporary resident in the US.

How Our Social Environment Plays Spoil Sport

It's not only women who are the recipient of snide remarks, but men also face direct attacks on their masculinity.

Deepan recounts his ordeal with his elder brother:

> I knew the worst was to come. My elder brother had his first child and there was celebration in the family. His painfully treacherous wink to me suggested that it was my turn now. In all this, our relationship suffered too. Quite anxiously my wife and I started on the path of trying to conceive but months passed by without any results. I felt emasculated. Within years, most of my friends had become parents, and at every gathering, eyes would be on us. 'Now it's time to slow down on your work and focus on having a family', we were told every time. We tried everything—improving our lifestyle, diet, everything but now it's been almost two years that we have been mechanically trying. Our family took notice too but at least they were nice to us. They tried to convince both of us that it was the right time for us to have a first baby. Annoyingly, my brother started getting on my case, too; he had had his second child by then. He counselled me that I was being selfish not thinking about a family although it had been five years since our marriage. He had a way of being intrusive, like asking me if my health was okay.[103]

---

103 Ibid.

The fear of ridicule is tougher for men because they can't easily emote, and thus, they take recourse to unhealthy habits like drinking. Our office culture is also not that evolved where you can talk about your infertility issues and request much-required leaves for clinic visits. This adds to workplace stress. And this stress continues to build up, which in turn can lead to further deterioration of sperm health.

Strained Relationships

All this takes a toll on the most important relationship—the husband-and-wife relationship. Men are sensitive towards their wives' needs but sometimes the wife puts too much pressure on him—the pressure to be her rock, the pressure to take the right decisions about the fertility treatment, dodging bullets from family and society, and empathetically handle her mood swings. All of this is justified expectation between the couple, but the wife must understand that infertility is new for men, too. They are equally anxious, scared and confused, but they are expected to behave in a certain way, meeting all the expectations from their end and being understanding, while their own emotional struggles get suppressed. We need to understand that men are also grappling in this blind alley of infertility.

In these cases, women need to be more resilient, sensitive to men, especially if the onus of infertility lies with the man. In our moments of grief, we are conditioned to think, 'Why me?' Reverse the thought process, be calmer, and take this as a part of life that shall pass, too.

Infertility is more complex because there are two people intrinsically involved in it. Thus, the relationship between a couple becomes more important here. The truth is that couples who go through infertility develop a much stronger bond because they form a team that fights together.

The rainbow has two ends; while on the one hand, there are men who support their wives and at least make an effort to understand and handhold, on the other end of spectrum, there are men who are a total waste of time.

One of our community members had to go through domestic violence when finally, after two years of dilly dallying, she could convince her husband for the sperm test, the result of which was azoospermia. The husband threatened to divorce her if this ever came out. Her in-laws, ignorant about the real cause, kept blaming the lady who had PCOS and was overweight for not being able to give them their *varis*. *Family tensions escalated and* had to undergo IVF knowing fully well that it would fail as the sperm issue wasn't even addressed.

In another case, the man couldn't stand up to his parents who were against IVF and putting the 'masculinity' of their son under the scanner. Finally, when the father-in-law passed away, the couple was able to go for IVF and they had a beautiful girl child; but they had to undergo sixteen years of stress and wait for this day.

The Myths

When infertility strikes, irrational thinking becomes a part of the coping process. Disturbing thoughts leave an indelible mark on your psyche, often jarring your self-esteem and causing a long-term repercussion. It is important to identify these traits, accept that these are myths and don't deserve your attention and that they need to be weeded out at the soonest.

Size of the penis and excessive masturbation has absolutely no connection with fertility. This is the most common myth that makes men feel low about themselves and becomes like a double question on your masculinity. Body shaming is for real. Be rest assured that this is a big myth with no medical standing. You have to get this out of your system.

When you are in India, you can't do away with myths arising out of religious and superstitious beliefs. One such dominant belief is that it is past karma that brings upon a curse like infertility. Falling for these beliefs and blaming yourself can only harm your physical and mental health.

Infertility is not a curse. It is just a medical condition that can be dealt with medically and psychologically, but you can never let it overwhelm you completely. Superstitious thoughts like these will not let you keep your sanity. You need a balanced body and mind to deal with a complicated issue like infertility. So, let go of these superstitions if you come across them. You must stop getting manipulated by society-led superstitions.

11
Managing Social Pressure

My Dear Unborn Child

I see you in our childhood pics
You may never resemble
In the baby showers and gifts
I may never have
I see you in the kid's dresses
I cannot buy
In the birthday parties
We may not get to celebrate
In baby toys which
May never be on my floor
In the tantrums and cries
I may never get to soothe
In your big kiddy problems
We may never get to solve
In your first steps, your first cycle ride

How to Get Pregnant with IVF

> *Your first fall and rubbed knee*
> *In the swings and commotion in the park nearby*
> *I see you all around me*
> *But not in my arms*
> *I long for your little hand to hold my finger*
> *Your tight hug, your little head on my shoulder,*
> *Your peaceful sleep, that says everything is alright*
> *I see you every month in the doctor's clinic*
> *I endure the injections, test and medicines month after month*
> *In the hope that someday I may really see you smile*
> *And run towards me and call me your mumma*
> *My child, you are not even born yet*
> *But you've held me for life*
> *Love, your yet to be mama and papa*[104]

Dharaa (pen name) is forty years old and lives in Noida. She is the author of this poem. She was once employed but is without a job now because she couldn't strike a balance between work and her infertility treatments. 'Thanks to the insensitive corporate laws', she says painfully.[105] After many failed IVF treatments and unsure thoughts about adoption, she fell into a deep depression. It is during this time that she wrote this touching poem.

---

104 Poem by Dharaa (pen name), Dharaa: Feelings in Ink, Dharaa.a, available at https://instagram.com/dharaa.a?igshid=YmMyMTA2M2Y=.

105 Interview with Dharaa, a forty-year-old woman, Noida.

Mandeep, a thirty-four-year-old from Delhi, who has been married for ten years, and has been trying to conceive for four years, says:

> At social gatherings, people ask you questions. It hurts but you can't do anything to stop them. By that time, I had withdrawn to an extent, but I had to listen. Some people genuinely care. It's not all wrong. But this is Indian society. Aunties are interested in other people's families. The younger generation is changing but that percentage is very small.[106]

Mithra Bindu, a thirty-nine-year-old from Kolkata who works as a freelance copywriter and whose husband is in the Indian Army, finally chose adoption post multiple IVF failures and unexplained fertility. She says:

> Sadly, God had other plans for me and from thereon started the longest battle of fifteen years! A battle of avoiding family members, ignoring friends and severing ties with society! I wanted to run away from society and from those baby questions which pierced my heart every time. Those questions which were telling me, 'Mithra, your planning has failed.'[107]

---

106 Interview with Mandeep, a thirty-four-year-old, Delhi.

107 Interview with Mithra Bindu, a thirty-nine-year-old freelance copywriter, Kolkata.

Social pressure is like a viral fever that catches you when you're low on immunity. As a woman going through infertility, you are low on emotional immunity and this is exactly the time when social pressure can knock you off your feet. The simplest way to ward off social pressure is to build your internal immunity and to make yourself emotionally stronger. Here are some ways you can do this:

Lose the Secretiveness

Often, we tend to hide things from people when they are rooted in shame, taboo, or they are things that are painful. Sometimes, we also hide our joys. Fighting infertility is all about courage and resilience. Society expects us to keep these issues a secret. Your family will ask you not to speak about them to anyone. Like with every major challenge, at the end of the day, the choice to tell people about your infertility issues is yours. I am not asking you to shout it from the rooftops, but in all my years of dealing with this and helping other women find light in this dark tunnel, I've realized that keeping it within you, maintaining the façade of normalcy, is more exhausting and directs energy away from your focus. Better still would be to accept the problem, speak about it matter-of-factly as you would for any other medical issue, thus setting a can-do building block approach to this journey.

Look the Predator in the Eye

If you think about it, our society is a bit like the animal kingdom. And the power dynamics remain the same. The stronger animal will bully the weaker one—chase, corner, and finally get them. The only way to stave off bullying is if the weaker animal holds its ground and shows its inner strength. This is the only way to make a bully step back. So, at a social gathering, if you feel threatened or bullied to answer questions about your pregnancy, answering the question head-on, matter-of-factly, will usually stop further questioning. Firm and honest—that's the way to go. For example, if an older relative is taking a jibe at you, 'When is the good news? Aren't you taking too much time?', instead of avoiding her and her question, tell her/him what you're going through, while leaving out the emotional aspect of it. You'll find that they either lose interest or start avoiding you so as not to receive such brutally honest answers which make them uncomfortable.

Stay in Your Herd

In the jungle, animals stay in similar groups to protect themselves from predators. For example, in Serengeti in Tanzania, you'll find that gazelles, zebras and buffaloes stick together because not only are they prey for lions, hyenas, etc., but there's also strength in numbers. And there's strength in community. Numbers and community give you strength because there are similar people going through similar issues who are, thus, empathetic towards your condition. You'll feel less alone. It is natural to feel drained fighting the world and infertility together but being in a group will help you recharge and draw positive energy. Join a support group, connect with women who have been through a similar journey, or are currently sailing in the same boat.

Anitha, a thirty-eight-year-old corporate managament professional from Chennai, and now a mother of two kids, told me that during her infertility journey, her closest confidant was her younger sister. She would talk to her often. Her sister was her rock. When Anitha opted for IVF, her sister had just gotten married. Despite that, she came and stayed with Anitha and chose not to get pregnant before her because if she did, then people would talk about Anitha.

Don't Get Intimidated

Your goal is clear. Don't get distracted. Excessive social pressure will derail you. Pressure in literal terms is simply a test. You need to give the test and come out with flying colours. Don't get intimidated by the test. Preparation is the key to managing social pressure test. Prepare well, stay strong, and you will come out a winner.

Choose Your Weapon

This is your journey. You need to build your strength to survive it. You need to choose your own way of handling the emotional and physical stress that comes along with it. There is nothing right or wrong about the method as long as it works for you and keeps the pressure off from your fertility journey.

Some women choose to be vulnerable. They will seek support, cry, show their desperation, and depend on the

Managing Social Pressure

validation of society. A woman showing weakness and being vulnerable is accepted in the Indian society as men believe that women are weaker and they become the protective spokespersons for these women. However, the downside is that they tend to become overbearing, and it might feel suffocating after a while.

Some women will choose to be reclusive. They will keep busy and avoid social gatherings or common interactions. They choose to be quiet and dignified. They won't give away any information and they diplomatically keep society confused.

Some women choose to tackle it head-on. They will be aggressive and ensure that the other party realizes that they have been hurt. They will simply cut off negativity. The downside in this is that you'll make more enemies, and then theses bruised egos will talk about you.

As I said at the onset, there is no right or wrong way of managing pressure. The goal is simple. You must keep the social pressure off in ways that best suit your personality, your family environment, and where you are in your fertility journey.

Dear Society, I am breaking up with you,
It's not me, but you who deceits me,
Dear Society,
I am breaking up with you
I abide by all your rules,
I did everything to please you, but still, you left me alone.
Dear Society,
I am breaking up with you

> *Now, you no longer own my body,*
> *You no longer own my thoughts*
> *But yes, you owe me a child*
> *Dear Society, am breaking up with you*
> *I am not going to smile at you,*
> *This time, it's going to be war*
> *The thin, pretty girl you trained,*
> *Followed your rules*
> *But not anymore,*
> *Dear Society,*
> *I am breaking up with you*
> *I hope you had fun*
> *But I am sure I won't miss you!*[108]

This short poem was anonymously shared on the Fertility Dost Facebook group by a young girl who diligently followed all the societal rules in the hope of having a child. She was alone, without a child, but she didn't let the fire inside her die. She chose not to be a victim but the master of her life.

Infertility is a traumatic experience which impacts the physical, financial and psychological wellbeing of a couple. The trauma of infertility doesn't start when you realize that baby-making isn't happening easily and naturally for you. In fact, the trauma begins much earlier—most women experiencing infertility now have had a history of PCOS, endometriosis, fibroids and period issues. They have been fighting reproductive health issues for a long time, and when

---

108 'Fertility Dost', Facebook, available at https://www.facebook.com/groups/fertilitydost.

it catapults into infertility, it becomes unbearable. Bearing pain and social stigma for so long is excruciatingly draining, to say the least.

Motherhood is so intrinsically connected to your womanhood that in a social sense you are not considered a complete woman if you are unable to procreate. In Tier 2 and below cities with a higher percentage of illiteracy and women still in the shackles of patriarchy, you will witness this blatant social stigma making life hell for a woman undergoing infertility. I met a young girl who was merely twenty-three or twenty-four years old. She was making a good number of eggs but wasn't able to conceive naturally. She was at an IVF centre, pleading with the doctor to do an IVF cycle for her. The doctor wasn't ready because all her reports were good, and this was no age to try for IVF. I was asked to counsel her. The girl meekly confessed that her mother-in-law has given her an ultimatum that if she doesn't bear a child by the end of the year, she will marry her son off to another girl. It turned out that the husband had infertility problems, but for the obvious reason of patriarchal protection, he didn't turn up for the test. The onus of having the baby fell singularly on the shoulders of this poor girl.

Girls are told to marry, have kids, and manage a perfect family, but as a woman when you find out that you can't have kids naturally, your social upbringing comes crashing down on you. It's not easy to break away from years of social conditioning and stereotyping. You can't do it overnight, and surely you can't do it when you are feeling ditched by the universe.

When it doesn't go the way that you have been taught or the way that you had planned it, the shock hits you, big time. Everything seems messed up and you feel completely lost in this new world of infertility.

Infertility is a medical condition. When you have a fever or jaundice, then you go to a doctor, get some medicines, take some rest, eat nutritious food, and people around you take care of you. But God forbid! If you have infertility, even accepting it as a problem is a big challenge. If it turns out that the problem is with the man, then it is another war to fight. All you can do is deflect and ignore.

Pain
You made me a, You made me a believer
Believer
Pain
You break me down, You build me up believer
Believer
Third things third, send a prayer to the ones up above
All the hate that you heard has turned your spirit to a dove

– 'Believer', song by Kurt Hugo Schneider, Will Champlin

Dealing with Stray Comments and Questions

'How can you be busy? You don't have kids.'

This is an example of the kind of statements that people might sometimes pass, without realizing that they could be hurtful or

Managing Social Pressure

demeaning to you. Not everyone will know what you're going through to always be sympathetic towards your emotional state. However, it is important that you learn to realize the difference between stray comments and actual bullying.

When I asked Anitha if she blamed herself for not getting pregnant, she instantly said yes. She would look at everyone in her family, her friends who had babies, and think what is so wrong with her that she couldn't get pregnant. Recalling her time during the procedure, she thinks that society's way of looking at women after marriage hasn't changed. If in a certain time frame post marriage you don't have children, society's attitude towards you changes. They start asking you in subtle ways. Having children should be a choice. It should not happen because your parents, in-laws or society say so. Because raising children is not an easy task.

Aiza is thirty-four years old. She's from Assam but lives and works in Gurugram. Aiza had two miscarriages and was contemplating IVF; she was not comfortable going everywhere because of the questions she was asked about her infertility. She told me,

> People will ask you: What is the problem? Why you are not conceiving even after five years of marriage? You don't want to answer but you have to respond. In a city like Gurgaon, it is still okay but when I go to my hometown in Assam you have to answer, and it is the worst thing in life. When I see my friends are having kids and they are playing around then I feel as

if I am only one deprived of this joy because of my own bad karma.[109]

Well-Meaning Advice from Relatives

In Indian families, relatives play a major role. They are first curious and then overbearing. They will push you to go to the clinic or healer of their recommendation, and if you don't relent, they tend to get offended. Your act of defiance is seen as rudeness as they were trying to help you.

Jaisanavi, a thirty-seven-year-old staying in Delhi, who left her career while undergoing the treatment, and so, is currently a homemaker, says:

> See, many people say many things. I mean my family is supportive. They trust my decisions on everything. But random people will give you advice such as go to this doctor, try this clinic, this treatment. But these are not my people; they're just some relative or acquaintance or a stranger. These things hurt because they don't know what we are going through, and how can they suggest things when they don't know what we have already tried? I've been on it since 2011. Not a single day has passed that I don't think about conceiving or trying to get pregnant. I am on it since a very long time. Every day I do something or the

---

109 Interview with Aiza, a thirty-four-year-old, Gurugram. Aiza is now a happy mother of a beautiful girl child.

other; try some remedy to conceive. I was asked to go to some baba in Ghaziabad. I was recommended to stop eating some things, to start eating some things. But just by eating or not eating something I don't think such a huge problem can be solved.[110]

Naina, a twenty-seven-year-old, married for almost five years and trying for a baby for the past three years with two spontaneous ectopic pregnancies, two failed IVFs and one cancelled frozen embryo transfer (FET), is inconsolable at this point in her life. She says:

From being a young, charming and a very dynamic girl who everyone talked about and wanted to be like, suddenly I became an under confident and silent girl. Standing in a group my only fear is being asked, 'So when are you giving us the good news?' Seeing friends having their first and now second babies is a feeling that can't be put in words. Going for baby showers or baby birthdays is a nightmare. I have lost a lot to this infertility fight in the last three years.[111]

Then these are the relatives who will be the first to tell you to step away from a ceremony because being 'childless' is inauspicious. That hurts. In every social gathering, the

---

110 Interview with Jaisanavi, a thirty-seven-year-old homemaker, Delhi.

111 Interview with Naina, a twenty-seven-year-old.

question of, 'So, when will you give us the good news?' will pop out. If you are a working woman, then it is a double attack. It is assumed that you are not bothered to have babies because you love your 'freedom'. These mean, below-the-belt comments, having fun at your cost, presumptions attitude, and the overall toxicity of the environment is stressful to handle, and you start avoiding family gatherings thereafter.

I have seen so many cases getting unnecessarily complicated by the unreasonable interference of in-laws. Sadly, if you have the wrong set of in-laws, there is no easy way out of this melodrama. Often, it is not what they say but how they say that is unsettling. You can't have a 'sex education talk with your MIL' at thirty years when the whole agenda of private talk is to impress upon how you are not doing sex enough or properly. It is surely an uncomfortable discussion, and you are sure to get offended. What follows is a huge drama by the MIL with the excuse that she was just being a good mom. And the vicious cycle of stress and complex relationships begins.

Rashi, a thirty-two-year-old resident of Gurugram who has been struggling with infertility for eight years, talks about her stressful experience with her in-laws when her younger brother-in-law had a baby. She says:

> People around me have been really supportive but my mother-in-law would indirectly say that in 2016 my brother-in-law got married and within a year,

they had a child. So, there were lot of differences being created between the two of us. We have been trying for a child for past eight years but haven't been able to succeed. Even my father-in-law mentioned it a couple of times that in his village there was this family who did not have kids, so the man went ahead for a second marriage.

I was too sad. I was so depressed that I have tried to hurt myself many a times and even asked my husband to go ahead with second marriage.[112]

Dr Sonia Malik, IVF doctor, Delhi, recounts how a father-in-law offered his sperm when a couple was diagnosed with male infertility and she had suggested donor sperm cycle as a solution. 'It was repulsive, deeply bred in patriarchy, unethical and immoral at so many levels. It is just wrong that a father-in-law would even offer to be a donor to keep the mythical genetic lineage intact', she says.

Dr Parul Katiyar, a senior IVF consultant, Delhi, cites a case where the father-in-law kept a tab on his daughter in law's menstrual cycle. While the father-in-law was over-involved during the consultation, the girl sat quiet and embarrassed. Not only was this a breach of her privacy, but also extremely humiliating.

As the in-laws of a sensitive couple struggling with infertility, you must be extra-emphatic, accommodating,

---

112 Interview with Rashi, a thirty-two-year-old, Gurugram.

and most importantly, trusting. It is known that what you are saying or doing is out of concern. It is also understood that in your times, infertility wasn't that big an issue and you don't have much clue about ART, except hearsay. So, instead of blurting out advice, try showing your concern genuinely by trying to first understand the situation holistically and giving advice when specifically asked for. Mostly importantly, give them space to process their thoughts. A woman just out of IVF failure doesn't need your advice. She simply needs the comfort of home, the love of her family, and a positive space to process her loss. Give her that space. Don't intrude or try to hasten the healing process. Trust that they are doing the best they can. Don't question their choices. They might seem irrational from where you are looking, but let them make their mistakes, let them figure this out themselves. At best, you can be an observer and comforter.

The good part is that all this will change soon. Once you cross over the fertility journey, you won't even remember or feel bad about it. During the fertility journey, we are living on the edge and become a bit too sensitive. Everything and anything can cause imbalance. It is quite natural for a person meeting you for the first time to ask about your family, marriage and kids. Usually, asking about kids is an icebreaker. However, the real problem is when the other person has some inkling about your situation, or is triggering you on purpose to get more information, or simply has negative vibes. It is best to avoid such people.

In Offices

I was working in a midsize company when I had my third miscarriage. The doctor asked me to rest for two to three weeks minimum. Work-from-home was not known back in those days. I had to ask HR for leave and when she asked the reason for such a long leave, I just spurted out something random. I didn't have the guts to tell her the truth for the fear of being judged and labelled. However, the worst was yet to come. I had to confide in my immediate boss (who was a woman) about my miscarriage and assumed that she would be empathetic. I walk into the office two weeks later. My boss asked me to come to a meeting room for a quick one-on-one chat. After the formal 'How are you?' pat came the question, 'So, what is your future plan? Will you try to conceive again? I mean I understand but giving such leaves will be difficult if these incidences happen on a frequent basis.'

Exasperated! I had no words to counter such insensitivity.

Yes, I will try to conceive again. Yes, I might require leave again. And, no I can't predict or plan the future, given my circumstance of fighting infertility; I answered by saying this with a lump in my throat.

Needless to say, this miscarriage leave was sugar-coated as a reason for not giving me a raise in the next appraisal.

Mandeep, a thirty-four-year-old from Delhi, is an MBA and was in a corporate job, but she quit because of her

IVF treatment. 'Work becomes difficult. There isn't enough flexibility for the treatment when you are working', she says.

Kasha, Assistant Professor in Computer Science, says, 'When you go for an IVF it takes about fifteen days for the procedure, you also need to rest for fifteen days. Who will give so many leaves? Due to this reason, I had to leave my job.'[113]

Being a woman acing the corporate ladder is tough in itself; you add to it the six months maternity benefit that raises eyebrows, now top it with infertility crisis and the myriad stigma attached to it; most offices in India are reluctant to have a conversation about the real issues. Women undergoing miscarriages or infertility have to ask for leaves under false pretext since the truth is a taboo, and if the management gets to know about their health condition, their career growth is at stake. So, everything is done discreetly. You have to be on alert all the time and not even let your colleagues know for the fear of being judged and tagged. All this hiding and being discreet adds to the stress of a couple who are already undergoing a traumatic journey.

Even in interviews, women are openly asked about their motherhood plans. I find this highly gendered and objectionable. Hire me for my skills and not to save your maternity benefit cost. Never join a company that asks this question in the interview, no matter how sugar-coated it is. This question is equivalent to asking for dowry in a marriage. You assess the family you are going into. Top

---

113 Interview with Kasha, Assistant Professor in Computer Science.

companies like Google, Facebook, and the likes have good HR practices in place to support women. Don't hesitate to ask your company HR about the policies.

According to Maternity Benefit Act, 1961, 'Leave for miscarriage. -- In case of miscarriage, a woman shall, on production of such proof as may be prescribed, be entitled to leave with wages at the rate of maternity benefit for a period of six weeks immediately following the day of her miscarriage.'[114]

According to the Maternity (Amendment) Bill, 2017, an amendment to the Maternity Benefit Act, 1961, passed by the President of India on 27 March 2017, a few additions keeping in mind the evolving environment have been added. These are:

> Maternity leave for adoptive and commissioning mothers—Maternity leave of 12 weeks to be available to mothers adopting a child below the age of three months from the date of adoption as well as to the 'commissioning mothers'. The commissioning mother has been defined as biological mother who uses her egg to create an embryo planted in any other woman.[115]

---

114 Maternity Benefit Act, 1961, available at https://labour.gov.in/sites/default/files/TheMaternityBenefitAct1961.pdf.

115 Maternity Benefit (Amendment) Act, 2017, Wikipedia: The Free Encyclopedia, available at https://en.wikipedia.org/wiki/Maternity_Benefit_(Amendment)_Act,_2017.

This Act is applicable to all organizations with ten or more employees and is available for all women working in the public and private sector. It also emphasizes that the employees are made fully aware of this policy in person and through email.

When you are going through IVF and have been asked by doctors to take bed rest, it is advisable to speak with the concerned person in office and avail work from home option. It is a win-win situation for both the parties. Otherwise, sadly, you have to fall back on your regular leaves and the mood of the reporting manager.

Society, on the whole, needs to build empathy towards a couple going through infertility.

Dear Society,

Please take a chill-pill. Stop questioning and judging, just hug her.

Social Media Pressure

Social media is now another convoluted tool for exerting social pressure. I asked a blogger friend to write about infertility and social taboos as a part of an awareness drive. While she aligns with the need to speak on such a relevant topic, she hesitated to openly express opinions on social media. It wasn't like her. She is Bengaluru-bred, works in a top MNC, and is a proactive-in-intellectual-conversations kind of a girl. I was intrigued. It turns out that she has decided to consciously go 'child-free' and she and her partner are trying to bring the family around to this decision. Now, if she actively talks about infertility on social media, her relatives will conclude that there is something wrong with her and that's why she is pushing to be 'child-free' to hide her infertility, and the unwanted sympathies will start pouring in.

Needless to say, how many times have we judged others for even liking or commenting a random post? 'Oh! She liked a post that talks about marital discord. I hope everything is fine between them'; thus goes the rounds of gossip driven by social media activities.

Then there is the issue of blatant or targeted marketing. A lady once recounted how, when she got pregnant, she joined all the pregnancy support groups, liked the baby product's pages, and subscribed to newsletters that tell you what to do at each stage of pregnancy. Sadly, she underwent a nasty miscarriage in her first trimester. While she was trying to recover from her traumatic loss, Facebook was at its best, showing her advertisements of baby products and telling her how her baby has now grown from a grain to a bean size inside her tummy.

She kept unsubscribing, unliking, but there seemed to be no end to this. It was a right-there-on-her-face kind of advertisement, a nasty reminder of her recent loss.

Box 11.1: Pro Tip

> There is a 'Hide Ad Topics' function which users can find by opening Settings, then Ads. You need to click on 'Hide Ad Topics', where you can select to remove ads related to parenting from your timeline. There are options to remove parenting ads for six months, one year, or permanently.

Source: Created by the author.

Then there are these viral challenges or dare campaigns that will keep popping on your feed, giving you major fear of missing out (FOMO). Motherhood dare was one such super-irritating campaign for our tribe of fertility warriors. One lady said that it is disturbing and makes her feel 'incomplete'. She decided to stay away from social media till the viral campaign exuberance dies down.

Make Your Partner Your Best Friend

This is the best way to fight social pressures. Make your partner your best friend in this journey. I don't know how much it will take for you to cross over the infertility bridge, but one thing I can say with complete certainty is that your relationship with your partner will evolve beautifully if both of you are in this together.

Misha Roderigues, a café owner from Goa who is in this fertility journey for the past five years and had an IVF failed recently, from my 'Fertility Dost' community, said when I asked her who is her best friend in this journey:

> No treatment so far is successful for us, but yes, the only good thing about this struggle is that it has brought us closer. My husband cannot stay hungry for long but on the day of my IVF pik up and transfer he was standing right outside the Operation Theatre until he saw me come back safe. It has to be a 50/50 partnership. Our husbands are managing their office, the finances, our moods, family, relatives, friends, medicines, driving us to the doctor's, even managing household chores as we are not in a state to do them. All without complaining.[116]

Mili Saxena, a twenty-five-year-old budding travel blogger from Udaipur, says:

> I never thought, husband can become best friend. While going through this infertility journey, hum kab best friend ban gaye pata hi nh chala ♥ [I didn't even realize when we became best friends]. Like in the last three years never did I went alone to the hospital, he was always by my side, while taking injections, jab roti hu toh chup karata hai [he calms me when I cry], or side mei jakar khud rota hai (but he himself cries hiding from me). Egg retrieval wale

---

[116] Interview with Misha Roderigues, a café owner, Goa.

din, meri pasand ka khana order karta hai, choti choti khushiyan ko celebrate karna 🎉 Pata hi nhi chala kab vo mera best friend ban gaya. My husband cum dost ♥ [my husband orders my favourite food on the egg retrieval day to cheer me up and takes care of all my small joys. He is my best friend].[117]

Some partners might not cooperate fully or show compassion openly, but you must continue to try and align them towards the common goal of parenthood. To become good parents, you should have a comfortable and understanding companionship. If someone tells you that have a baby and the presence of baby will solve all your marital relationship issues then don't plan a baby for this reason. It will simply worsen the situation.

Inspiration from Mythology

Infertility is nothing new, and our Gods and Goddess have been through it, and frankly they were much more open to alternative solutions than we are.

As a child, we all grew up listening to stories of Kunti, the wife of Pandu who gave birth to five sons and all were supposedly born miraculously. We were made to believe that she stood in the balcony, closed her eyes, meditated

---

[117] Interview with Mili Saxena, a twenty-five-year-old budding travel blogger, Udaipur.

on a certain God, uttered some mantra, and lo and behold! The next minute she had a baby in hand. Is this some kind of magic? Are these fictitious stories? When you are a child, these make perfect sense. But when you outgrow that stage, you realize that babies cannot be created through mantras. What we didn't know then is that Kunti's was a classic case of artificial insemination where a donor sperm was used to inseminate her because her husband Pandu was supposedly impotent. However, the truth behind these stories is well hidden and one needs to dig deeper to understand what lies beneath the surface.

Our dear Lord Krishna is an inspiring example of the beauty of adoption. It is universally known that he was brought up not by his biological parents, but by his adoptive parents. This means that adoption was neither unknown nor unacceptable back in those days. His mother adoption, Yashoda, is certainly more revered than his birth mom, Devaki.

Consider Gandhari. Is it humanly possible for someone to give birth to 100 sons? Well! Logically, no. Then what explains the birth of the Kauravas? Some say that it is a kind of IVF where Gandhari gave birth to a grey mass which was cut by Sage Vyasa into 100 pieces and kept in a pot immersed in ghee to incubate. A year later, each grew to be a son. It is possible that Vyasa had knowledge of advanced IVF, which helped fertilize the children outside Gandhari's womb.

Inspiration from Celebrities

'Here I was at the age of twenty-three being told that I would never conceive. I was shattered', said Nita Ambani, Indian philanthropist and wife of industrialist Mukesh Ambani.[118] At twenty-three, she was diagnosed with infertility. 'My parents had us after seven years of marriage—my twin Akash and I were IVF babies', Isha Ambani, daughter of Mukesh and Nita Ambani, said in a *Vogue* interview in 2019.[119]

Ace choreographer Farah Khan Kunder hit the headlines in 2008 when she gave birth to triplets through IVF. According to her, 'When the choice is to either go childless or IVF, there is no room for doubts. I was forty-three when I had my kids and my biological clock had stopped ticking long time ago.'[120] She made her choice public at a time when infertility issues were still a taboo and shoved under the

---

[118] TNN, 'At 23, Nita Ambani was told that She Could Never Conceive', ETimes, 18 April 2019, available at https://timesofindia.indiatimes.com/life-style/parenting/pregnancy/at-23-nita-ambani-was-told-that-she-could-never-conceive/articleshow/68864007.cms.

[119] Priya Tanna, 'Exclusive: Isha Ambani Piramal on Work, Legacy and Life After Marriage', Vogue, 31 January 2019, available at https://www.vogue.in/content/isha-ambani-on-reliance-jio-marriage-exclusive-vogue-india-february-2019-cover-story.

[120] 'Bollywood Celebrities Who Did Not Conceive Naturally', Yahoo! News, 19 June 2013, available at https://sg.news.yahoo.com/bollywood-celebrities-did-not-conceive-naturally-055701366.html.

carpet. Today, Farah Khan is an inspiration to many women across the country to come out in the open about fertility issues.

After a miscarriage in 2009, Aamir Khan and Kiran Rao welcomed their son Azad in 2011 through IVF surrogacy. It was no mean task and gossip mills were churning vigorously on this juicy piece of byte. Aamir was quite open about it and declared, 'This baby is especially dear to us because he was born to us after a long wait and some difficulty.'[121]

After several years of the birth of their two kids, Shahrukh and Gauri Kham opted for IVF surrogacy when they planned for their third child. There was a lot of speculation, and for a long time, this was kept under wraps. Finally, Shahrukh confirmed, 'Amidst all the noise that has been going around, the sweetest is the one made by our newborn baby, AbRam.'[122]

Sohail and Seema Khan battled secondary infertility for ten years. The couple opted for IVF surrogacy in 2011, ten years after the birth of their first son. Secondary infertility is more common than we know. This Bollywood celebrity couple chose IVF surrogacy to have their second child and move on with their lives.

---

121 Ibid.

122 PTI, 'SRK Brings Baby AbRam Home, Denies Sex Determination Test', The Times of India, 9 July 2013, available at https://timesofindia.indiatimes.com/city/mumbai/srk-brings-baby-abram-home-denies-sex-determination-test/articleshow/20990413.cms.

Socialite Haseena Jethmalani and her husband, prominent lawyer Mahesh Jethmalani, had their twins ten years after the birth of their first daughter. Haseena was fifty at that time (in 2006) and proudly declared, 'I think IVF is one of the ways forward for women but most people shy away from it as unfortunately there is a certain stigma attached to being infertile.'[123]

Recently, Bollywood actresses Priyanka Chopra and Shilpa Shetty chose surrogacy, and each has a girl child through it.[124]

How to be a Good Friend?

I got a call from a very young, unmarried girl in her twenties, inquiring about how I can help in cases of infertility. I was surprised because she was so young. At first, I tried to figure out if she genuinely had a fertility problem or if it was a spam call. Soon, she told me that she was trying to help her colleague who she thinks is going through infertility, and while she really wants to help her, she couldn't figure out how. She didn't know how to broach the subject without

---

123 Sheela Das, 'Celebrity Couples Who Had Babies through IVF', Bollywood Mantra, 19 August 2016, available at https://www.bollywoodmantra.com/news/celebrity-couples-who-had-babies-through-ivf/23056/.

124 '20+ Indian Celebrities Who Chose IVF: The 'Un-Traditional Way'—2022', Fertility Dost, available at https://www.fertilitydost.com/articles/article-details/10-indian-celebrities-who-chose-ivf--the-un-traditional-way--2018.

seeming inappropriate or intrusive, which could affect their friendship. This was a tricky situation to handle. The line between being genuinely concerned and being inappropriately curious is very thin. However, I was happy that this woman going through infertility has such a good friend. Our society needs more such good friends.

One of the main points to remember before helping a friend who is undergoing the process of fertilization is to not give any gyaan (knowledge/wisdom). The couple is already confused and scared with varied guidance by experts in their family, friends and doctors. You don't want to add to it. Hence, giving a patient hearing and giving them the space to think on their own is a great way to mentally give them the strength to fight the bad/unwanted thoughts.

Second, be very careful while raising the subject with the couple. And do not so this without their consent. You need to earn their trust with small gestures, such as paying them a visit, listening to them and taking care of them. It is a very private aspect of life, and most couples prefer to keep the entire process of childbirth under wraps. Also, they're probably going through so much pressure that they may not feel inclined to share. Being in touch with the couple and just being there for them will help build trust. And it is crucial that as a friend you do not reveal or share their personal treatment-related information or discuss about them with anyone else without their permission.

Third, don't force or rush the couple into taking any action. The process of infertility to fertility is very exhaustive and needs to be nurtured and nourished with time and love. Hand-holding with one step at a time is quite helpful.

The fourth aspect is to not give advice or expert opinions to them over the phone. A personal touch of holding their hand heals the pain in a greater way. Avoid WhatsApp or texting; instead, hear them. The best way is to have a face-to-face dialogue. The gravity of the situation is very delicate, and it can make things good or worse for many.

Anuradha, a twenty-eight-year-old marketing consultant from Meerut, said poignantly when in her 'trying-to-conceive-phase':

> I am not going to lose myself to this beast called infertility. I am not letting *you* be *me*. Because I am Me, a topper in school, a gold medallist in college, a creative designer, a good wife, a good daughter and a good human being. I am not going to let you make me feel jealous when I see a pregnant lady or when I see a newborn. I am not going to let you make me feel incomplete. I am not going to let you stop me from laughing or attending baby showers. I am not going to let you make me miss life because I am much more than you. I am Me. Definitely not just an IVFer.[125]

---

125 Interview with Anuradha, a twenty-eight-year-old marketing consultant.

12

When to Stop
The Road Ahead

You gave it your best, you gave it your youth, now don't make it about your ego. Let it go, let it go…

I WAS TOTALLY LOST AFTER MY FIRST IVF FAILURE. I DIDN'T have the strength to go for the next cycle. After taking a break for a whole year from the treatment, I decided to do the second and the last IVF cycle with a clear resolve that if the second IVF would be positive, then absolutely fantastic; however, if it fails, then I would start the process of adoption right away without wasting another day sulking over my kismet (luck).And then there are couples who endure twenty-one IVF cycles to get pregnant. Such is the junoon (passion), as we call it.

Prakriti, a twenty-seven-year-old homemaker from Ujjain, recounts how family pressure made her reconsider and go for yet another IVF cycle: 'There was some pressure from the family to try again. We thought, okay, why not one more time. Ek aur baar sahi [let's try one more time].'[126] We live in a big joint family, and though I was neither prepared emotionally nor convinced, I didn't want to sound selfish when the whole family was rooting for my success. However, the IVF failed despite all the support, and I realized I wasn't being selfish but stupid.

Knowing when to stop or doing course correction is crucial. This is the most difficult phase of the journey. You have been through a lot of treatments, ups and down, failures, and maybe a few temporary successes. Your body feels like it has given up, your mind is a haze of confusion; it is like you are driving in the dark, not knowing when you will reach the destination. There may be a quietness in your relationship, and financially you must have stretched yourself to the maximum. Life seems to have completely slipped out of your control. All your plans have fallen flat, and this phase is simply out of syllabus.

Personally, I would say three rounds of IVF are more than enough, post which it is time to take a conscious call to move ahead. After three full rounds of IVF (stimulation cycles), you are just mindlessly following the protocol. How much can your body take? The signs begin to show, and there are side-effects, which we naively ignore because we have been taught that to become a mother you must endure pain.

---

[126] Interview with Prakriti, a twenty-seven-year-old homemaker, Ujjain.

Dr Munjaal says that their clinic's protocol is that they don't do IVF beyond six stimulation cycles (not counting the frozen cycles or surrogacy). Similarly, in the Indian Defence hospitals, IVF is capped at a maximum of four cycles. Needless to say, unethical clinics will use the carrot dangling methodology and keep luring you for more rounds.

This journey is full of internal conflicts.

Now is the time to think deeply about the most important question with an open mind…

Why do you want a child?

Whenever I ask this question to a woman trying to conceive, within a blink of an eye, answers will look something like this:

1. Is that even a question? Isn't everyone at my age expected to have a child?
2. I have been married for so many years; it is high time I have a child.
3. My husband wants to have a child.
4. My mother-in-law (or any close relative) is unwell and they desire to see my child at the soonest.

So, I ask them again: Why do *you* want to have a child?

You will think you know the answer, but you need to introspect deeper. The answers will come gradually. You may be surprised to find that that the reasons you wanted a child were influenced by society's expectations, stereotypes, prejudices, peer pressure, and your own idea of an ideal family.

If your answer is pure and simple, 'I want a child to raise a good human being on whom I want to shower my unconditional love', then you know you have reached the right thought process.

These were my reasons for having a child. At first, I wanted a child because everyone has a child after one year of marriage. When my first child is three years old, I can go back to my career. So, I just want to check this box as done and dusted. Then, I wanted a child because all my friends had one. I didn't get invited to birthday parties. Everyone in my circle was talking about diapers, baby food and stuff like that, and I had no inputs. I wanted to be a part of these mommy groups and circles.

Then I moved on to the stage where I was in a mad competition with my kismet, thinking:

> How the fuck can't I have a child? What's wrong with me? I will prove it to the world that I can have a child. I will hold it like a trophy and declare to this insensitive world that whatever you guys have been saying to me, I will prove you all wrong.

After my failures, I was begging to God, 'Give me a child. I will do whatever you want. I am Bengali but I will stop eating fish. I will not leave your temple till you give me a positive sign that you have listened to my plea.' Then came the stage of dignity:

Give me the strength to deal with this phase and to accept whatever you have decided for me. I want to have a child because I know I have an ocean of love bottled inside me and I just want to let loose, love unconditionally and mould a being into a beautiful human.

When I was at my wit's end with the fertility journey and was moving towards the final decision, there were two strong feelings that needed to be worked upon:

1. Have I given my best?
2. And closure.

Closure

Closure is important to let you move on.

Since my case was that of unexplained infertility, it was important for me to get closure. This answer would eventually put an end to my next question: 'Did I do enough?'

I had this feeling that I didn't give my best during the first IVF. So, I pushed myself in the second round, even though medically I was told not to risk another attempt of pregnancy and my family wanted me to go for adoption. The problem was that I didn't want to go for adoption with any lingering doubts. I couldn't lie to myself. My mind was constantly troubled with finding closure.

I decided to risk a second IVF attempt but with the promise that I would do whatever it took and give my best, and second, with mindful consciousness that this would be my final round. If I didn't succeed, I would move on knowing that I had left no stone unturned. It would be a fresh start thereon.

Every day, you will want to give up, and then you will hear a miracle story and want to continue. Your heart will urge you to push yourself. You will be plagued by doubt. What if the next round of IVF is a success? So and so had a child on her fourth IVF. I can't give up on my second.

Bindu, a thirty-nine-year-old, originally from Mumbai and now settled in US, who had eight long years of struggle with infertility and is now mother of two, Maya and Mukund, says:

> A 'no' that has a logical reason for not happening is much more comforting than a blanket 'no' without any explanation. We were going through the same thing when the doctors in the US made it clear that we can't conceive but they couldn't tell us 'WHY', We had come to an end, but without closure! I was not mentally ready for adoption. I was still hoping to get pregnant because our infertility was unexplained. This hide-and-seek game had lasted for eight years before it ended, and thankfully, it did end when I choose adoption. Being a mother has been the best part of my life. The road to being a mom was long, but I forgot the pain and the disappointment of

When to Stop

> multiple IVF failures when I said yes to adoption. I got my sense of relief and life back![127]

Moving on is a very personal decision and will depend on many factors. But primarily, it will be based on your interpersonal relationships, mindset, current state of emotional wellbeing, family background, and your experience with fertility journey. You will want to move on when:

1. You have exhausted all options that medical science has to offer.
2. You are not emotionally prepared for aggressive solutions like donor cycles.
3. You have a medical issue (such as azoospermia or physiological problems with the uterus) that can't be resolved.
4. You have found your closure and made peace with it.

These are some of the main parameters that can help you decide when to stop.

There are no easy answers or an easy path to this. It feels quite similar to being asked to unplug the ventilator of your loved one. He may or may not survive; most probabilities are pointing towards non-survival. You mind knows that he won't survive. Your heart wants to hold on to as long

---

127 Interview with Bindu, a thirty-nine-year-old, US.

as possible. Trust me, this will be one of the most difficult decisions of your life.

What Next?

When I ask couples this question, these are some of their initial responses:

1. We have accepted our fate of being childless.
2. We will travel and enjoy our life with each other.
3. We will remain childfree or be a Double Income No Kids (DINK)couple.

These answers are fine but let me tell you why these won't work in the long run. In the first statement, there is a sense of dejected resignation, a sense of remorse and a painful sting. This emptiness will keep pinching you for you never had proper closure, a logically resonating one.

The next statement is the by-product of delusional attitude. It shows that you haven't accepted it fully yet and are lying to yourself. You have always dreamt of travelling and enjoying your time together as a complete family. At a later stage, you might miss the feeling of a complete family.

In the third statement, the problem is that you should decide to remain childfree at the beginning itself, not post the fertility journey when it ceases to be a free choice, but rather, becomes a helpless option. You can't and shouldn't stay in denial forever.

I know it is difficult and painful but one must think of moving ahead and in the right direction. Don't make it a personal ego issue or some kind of competition where having a biological child will get you the winner status. Think with an open mind. If a child is what you want and for the right reasons, then adoption is a great way forward.

Adoption—The Heart Babies

Purnima, a woman in her thirties from Gurugram, had three failed IVFs and a fourth that partially succeeded; she had a stillborn twin pregnancy that left her totally devastated. 'It is not easy to see your baby die after six months of being pregnant, minutes after being born right there on the hospital bed', she says.

> I wanted to move on and pull myself out of my sorrow. I couldn't deal with it anymore, not try any longer because it had been a traumatic journey and if anything wrong happened now, I had no energy to deal with it. It's not like I did not want a child, I wanted a child, but I couldn't give birth to one. I decided to stop right there seeing the still born twins. The very next day I went for adoption and my whole family supported.[128]

Today, she is a happy mom of a teenage girl born out of her heart.

---

[128] Interview with Purnima, a woman in her thirties, Gurugram.

It is sad but true that adoption is the second option. There are only very few people who go for altruistic adoption. Most couples will begin thinking about adoption when the natural birthing process fails. If you are at a similar crossroads, be assured that it is not unconventional or unheard of. All you need to focus on now is to be fully prepared before going for adoption. You can't take this decision in haste as it is a child's life at stake here.

I was once advised by a well-meaning relative to adopt a child, and then the adopted child will bring happiness, which will help me conceive the second child naturally, and later, I can conveniently neglect the adopted child as now I have the biological one—a hack that sounded wrong at so many levels. There is no dearth of such Bollywood-inspired adoption theories. You must be unyielding to all these pressures and be fully prepared before advancing for adoption.

Mental Preparation is Key

'Adoption is always at the back of my mind but my husband is not yet convinced', confides Aiza from Assam.[129]

Be sure to go for adoption for the right reasons. Remember, it is all about acceptance and not adjustment. You aren't doing any social service by bringing a child home and giving her/him a home. On the contrary, the child is giving you a complete family. S/he is filling the void that you have in your current life.

---

129 Interview with Aiza, Assam.

When to Stop

Couples should first sit and have a clear conversation with each other. Thereafter, they should involve the immediate family, parents and siblings in this conversation. The couple should be informed and be on the same page for the adoption process and the journey afterwards to be smooth. Talk to an adoption counsellor if you are facing any challenges in communication with your husband or parents. Read the success stories and meet parents in adoption to crease out any understanding gaps.

When my first IVF failed, I initiated a conversation about adoption with my husband to get his opinion on the subject. We had a couple in our friends circle who had a very smart kid. Soumen, my husband, said that she is smart because her father is a doctor, concluding that genes play an important role in making a good child. I conceded because truly she was an ideal kid that any parent can dream of! A few years and a couple of miscarriages later, when I was going through a really bad time, the same doctor couple invited us for dinner to their home. It was then that seeing our distress, the lady said that she wanted to share something personal. She recounted her personal journey with infertility and how their daughter was adopted. It was a facepalm moment! Apparently, genes are not everything. My respect for them doubled and my myths about adoption disappeared.

It is the environment that you give the child that will shape everything, and not the genes. If genes were everything, kids of all scientists would have super IQ and no kid of a doctor would ever commit suicide. Stop thinking about this mythical element called 'genes'.

It is only natural that the subject of genes will play on your mind once you think about adoption. This is how a social stereotype is built and you can't do away with it overnight. All you can do is be clear between you and your partner about the decision and try to explain it to your immediate family.

The Process of Adoption

'Biology is the least of what makes someone a mother', Oprah Winfrey once said.

In India, the process of adoption is completely streamlined, legalized and parent-friendly, carried out through the Central Adoption Resource Authority (CARA). CARA is a government body that is the nodal agency for adoption.

As of January 2022, 36,000 couples are in queue waiting and CARA has only 1,936 kids for adoption.[130] If you want to go for adoption, don't delay anymore as already the waiting time is long.

Step 1: Submit Documents on the CARA Website

Just go to the CARA website, register, upload your documents, and fill the form as required, and you are done.

---

[130] Ambika Pandit, '36,000 Couples in Queue, But CARA has 1,936 Kids', The Times of India, 1 January 2022, available at https://timesofindia.indiatimes.com/india/36000-couples-in-queue-but-cara-has-1936-kids-report/articleshow/88625272.cms.

Yes! It is that simple. There is a list of documents on the CARA website. You get thirty days after starting to fill your form to collect and upload all the documents.

A few important pointers to remember while filling form are:

Age Bracket of the Baby You Opt for

There are age brackets of baby that you wish to adopt, starting from zero to two years, two to four years, following a similar two years of bracket till the eighteen years. So, you can adopt a child from zero to eighteen years. A couple's age should be ninety or less than ninety to opt for kids in the zero to two years age category. If your combined age (age of both the parents) is more than ninety years, you can only opt for a baby in the two to four years and above category. If the combined age of the parents is above 105 years, you can opt for the four to six years and above category. The other factor to consider is the waiting period. The maximum waiting period is for babies in the age group of zero to two years and two to four years. Out of 1,936 kids (as of January 2022) ready for adoption, only 3 per cent[131] are healthy and below two years (the category most sought after by couples desirous of adopting), which is roughly sixty-one kids, while there are approximately 24 per cent (approximately 463)

---

131 'Children Availability', Families of Joy Foundation, available at https://familiesofjoy.org/adoption-help-resources/children-available-for-adoption/.

children above the age of two years. Do the math yourself and choose the age group wisely.

Category

There are two categories of children—normal and special kids. You can opt for the category after giving it some thought and deciding on your personal preference. For obvious reasons, the waiting period for special children is comparatively lesser.

State Preference

You can choose to adopt from a particular state (any three states) or from anywhere in India. In case you select the option 'National' in the form then be prepared to travel to that particular city (anywhere in India) when you get the call. For ease and convenience, people often chose the regional centre.

You are asked to submit your and partner's latest photograph. This helps them match the physical attributes as much as they can. CARA tries their best to find the right match.

Step 2: Prepare for Home Visit

Once you have filled the form, you are asked to select your preferred location for the home study. This home visit is done by the Specialized Adoption Agency (SAA). You will get the complete contact details of the agency. You should

When to Stop

then coordinate with them for scheduling the home visit. This visit is not a surprise visit.

Within thirty days of document submission, your home visit will be scheduled. In the home visit, authorized people from CARA will come and visit your house. They will meet everyone who resides in the house, closely see around the house, ask a few questions, check your original documents, and based on this visit, they will prepare a report. It is best to ask them what original documents they need so that you can keep them handy. Also, they will require *two referral letters*. These referral letters can't be from any relatives. They must be provided by a friend, colleague or neighbour. This letter is to show that they know the couple well and that they are good people.

Another thing to be submitted is the *takeover letter*; this can't be given by the parents of either partner. They must be a sibling of yours. This is basically to assure who will take care of the kid in case of any eventuality with the parents. It can't be your parents as they are ageing and not logically capable for taking care of the kid.

At this stage, you have to pay Rs 6,000 as the agency processing fees.

The objective of this visit is to see the environment in which you plan to bring the baby and also to assess your and your family's emotional preparedness towards adoption. Just be yourself, stay normal, and answer honestly.

The only way you get a bad report is if you are still in two minds about adoption or someone who stays with you, say your parents, are not very convinced and show some resistance. The officials are trained for this job and they will sense if something is amiss.

This report is provided within thirty days. Thereafter, you will get the login id and username, and now officially you have moved on to the next stage.

Step 3: Waiting Period

Once you get an okay report from the home visit, the document phase stands complete. Now you are in queue. You can check your status online. It is completely transparent. The wait is usually two to two-and-a-half years for adoption of babies from zero to two years. If you have opted to adopt a child in the age bracket of two to four years, the queue is much shorter.

Mithra, a forty-year-old parent-by-adoption from Delhi, reminisces about her adoption waiting period: 'I think of how supportive my husband has been throughout the "waiting" years, handling the adoption paperwork and me, patiently.'[132]

Step 4: You have Your Child

Once you advance in the queue, you will begin to get child referrals. A child's photograph and basic details will pop up on your screen. You have to accept or decline. If you decline, you are shown another child. You only get a maximum of

---

132 Interview with Mithra, a forty-year-old parent-by-adoption, Delhi.

three chances. If you consume all three chances and are unable to make up your mind, sadly you will be pushed back to the end of the serpentine queue. So, be very careful at this stage and decline only if you have a very strong reason. Usually, people accept the first choice itself.

Now, there is another shortcut and that is called immediate placement (IP).

These are the kids who have been rejected five times by other parents. CARA aims at finding them a suitable home soon. You will see their details as a ticker on your screen. If you select them, irrespective of your queue status, you are called for immediate adoption. Mostly these are kids who are siblings. CARA, for ethical reasons, is against separating siblings. Sibling sets constitute of as many as 8 per cent of all children ready for adoption. Many parents don't want two kids together, so they decline; but if you are up for it, go ahead and jump the queue and bring double the happiness. They are absolutely normal kids.

*This is reflective as of January 2022, and the database is dynamic and keeps changing frequently. Please see the CARA website for the complete and latest database (available at http://cara.nic.in/).

Step 5: Go to the Adoption Centre to Meet Your Baby

Once you have selected the child, you have to immediately go to the adoption centre where you can physically meet the child. The centre might once again verify all your documents and give you a counselling session. The centre will give you medical reports and all the available details about the child. You can get the medical reports checked by your own doctor or even get a fresh set of tests conducted by your own doctor for complete assurance. You stay with the child for two to three days. Post all the documentation, you are ready to bring the child to your house.

At this stage, you have to pay Rs 40,000 as adoption processing fees.

Step 6: Signing Legal Documents

There is a period of ninety days when you and the child live together before the legal documentation is signed in court. All the legal processes are initiated by the adoption centre. You are called on a particular date to come with the kid and sign the adoption deed in court.

Post-Adoption Process

For the first year, you must bring the child twice at an interval of six months to the adoption centre so that they can make sure that the child is taken care of properly.

That's it. Enjoy this new phase of your parenthood.

Busting Myths

Older Kids Don't Bond Well

The kids in adoption centres are constantly counselled and prepared. They are eagerly looking forward to being adopted and know what adoption is much more than any of you would. They are much more mature and sensitive. All they need is love, and they will bond sooner and stronger than you would know. You must also approach without any preconceived notion.

When the Child Finds Out that They are Adopted They Might Just Leave Us

Real life is no Bollywood movie wherein everyone hides this taboo word 'adoption', and then one fine day, amidst hush-hush conversations, the child comes to know. Devastated, the child runs away to find her real parents. Nope.

You only hide things you are ashamed of, right? And surely you are not ashamed of the adoption that has given you so much joy. That's the perspective with which you have to approach this. A friend of mine who has adopted two daughters had told her elder daughter about her being adopted when she was as young as eight years.

Purnima shared how she had told her daughter about adoption. She was in a life-coaching workshop when she asked the psychologist on the panel how she could go about telling her daughter that she had been adopted. The psychologist said as a mother she will never have the strength to tell her and she will keep procrastinating, but you must tell the child for her emotional wellbeing. Purnima went back home, gathered all the strength she had, every ounce of it, held her fourteen-year-old daughter's hand, and told her the big truth with tears rolling down. The child shouted, screamed, locked herself in a room, kept crying, and didn't speak for three days. Purnima says that those were the toughest three days of her life. Purnima waited patiently. Finally, her daughter came out of the room and hugged her mother tight and said, 'You are my mother and will always be, just promise me that you will never leave me, never ever.'

Now this mother-daughter duo is the biggest champion of adoption. Nothing to hide, nothing to be scared of. Pure love.

What if the Child has a Medical or Learning Disability Issue that We Learn about a Few Years Later?

There are about 1,265 children with special needs looking for parents out of a total 1,936, as of January 2022 in India.[133] If you choose to adopt a special needs child, you can jump the long waiting queue.

Once you bring the child home and make her/him a piece of your heart, don't worry, you will overcome any challenges that might come. However, thorough medical and other tests are done by CARA and a detailed report is provided to you, which you can get cross-checked by a doctor of your own choice before you adopt the child. CARA ensures complete transparency in this regard. A disability at a later stage is highly unlikely.

---

133 'Children Availability', Families of Joy Foundation.

How Will I Breastfeed an Adopted Baby?

Yes, you can breastfeed your adopted child. There are medicines that can help you lactate, if you start taking them a few months ahead. If you plan properly, you can enjoy all the elements of motherhood, even the most intimate bonding moment, breastfeeding. Consult a lactation expert.

'Acceptance is the greatest reward we can give to ourselves. We can't control our lives, but we surely can control our attitude towards life. At the end of the day, it is how we survive our challenges that matters most', says Dr Malvika Iyer, Bomb blast survivor, President awardee, motivational speaker, and disability activist.[134]

---

134 Dr Malvika Iyer, @MalvikaIyer, Twitter, available at https://twitter.com/malvikaiyer.

Acknowledgements

Special thanks to my Fertility Dost community for inspiring me to write this book. The idea of the book started taking shape when I saw most of the couples in my community asking almost similar types of questions and struggling with more or less similar issues during this journey. They opened their hearts to me and spoke uninhibited, delving deep into the darkest, and often saddest phase of their life with one clear motive: if their story and learnings can help other couples find their way in this maze of infertility, it is all worth the effort. I am thankful to all those brave fertility warriors often looming in shadows and staying anonymous but leaving an indelible mark which transformed into the spirit and essence of this book.

My wonderful team at Fertility Dost supported and motivated me throughout this journey, especially when I was losing it all, juggling between writing the book, scaling up Fertility Dost and managing home. A small message from them, that we are eagerly waiting for your book to publish, would push me to burn the midnight oil. Purnima Sood, my team member, Co-Founder at Fertility Dost and my friend, would say, '*sab ho jayega* [everything will fall in place'] in her quintessential calming tone, and infuse me with the energy to keep going.

I would like to thank Sonal (former editor with HarperCollins) who tracked me on social media for a year before approaching me over an email, which I initially thought was a hoax! We met over coffee and bonded instantly. She sowed the seeds. Then came Trisha Bora, my editor, who ensured that I stick to timelines and pulled me out of procrastination.

I owe this book to my parents, Shekhar Chakrabarty and Renu Chakrabarty, who supported me unconditionally throughout my infertility struggle days. Their love, trust and pride for me gives me strength to break all the glass ceilings. And, not to forget my sister, Sonali Chakrabarty Singh, who shows her love and support in the weirdest and most unexpected ways. I am overwhelmed with the support and love of my in-laws and friends who kept me motivated and focused.

I am specially thankful to all the doctors who took out time from their busy schedules to help me with the medical inputs while I was researching for the book. They have believed in my mission throughout and have cheered me all along.

I am grateful to my co-fertility struggler, my life partner, my friend, and my ultimate punching bag, Col Soumendra Banerjee, for keeping me mostly sane. Hugs and love from Athindra Banerjee, my son, complete me. He is the reason I do what I do, and I am indebted to God for giving me such a beautiful reason to live.

About the Author

Gitanjali Banerjee is a journalist and the founder of Fertility Dost, an online infertility support group that has over 50,000 members. She struggled with infertility for almost a decade before conceiving through IVF.

30 Years *of*
HarperCollins *Publishers* India

At HarperCollins, we believe in telling the best stories and finding the widest possible readership for our books in every format possible. We started publishing 30 years ago; a great deal has changed since then, but what has remained constant is the passion with which our authors write their books, the love with which readers receive them, and the sheer joy and excitement that we as publishers feel in being a part of the publishing process.

Over the years, we've had the pleasure of publishing some of the finest writing from the subcontinent and around the world, and some of the biggest bestsellers in India's publishing history. Our books and authors have won a phenomenal range of awards, and we ourselves have been named Publisher of the Year the greatest number of times. But nothing has meant more to us than the fact that millions of people have read the books we published, and somewhere, a book of ours might have made a difference.

As we step into our fourth decade, we go back to that one word – a word which has been a driving force for us all these years.

Read.

    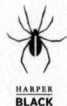 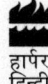